Cocaine use is dangerous. It is also illegal unless prescribed by a physician. However, its use and abuse are realities in our society. As publishers of *The Coke Book*, we are not in favor of cocaine use, but we believe it is our responsibility to disseminate as much information as we can to the widest possible public about this controversial subject. We offer this book in the hope that it will bring clarity and factual information to the growing public debate about cocaine.

THE COKE BOOK

THE COMPLETE REFERENCE TO THE USES AND ABUSES OF COCAINE

BERT STERN
Producer

LAWRENCE D. CHILNICK
Editor-in-chief

TEXT BY

R.C. GARRETT
U.G. WALDMEYER
VIVIENNE SERNAQUE

MEDICAL CONSULTANTS

DAVID E. SMITH, M.D.
Medical Director/Founder, Haight-Ashbury Free Medical Clinic, San Francisco

RICHARD B. SEYMOUR, M.A.
Director of Training, Haight-Ashbury Free Medical Clinic, San Francisco

---

RESEARCH AND PRODUCTION

DANIEL MONTOPOLI

BERKLEY BOOKS, NEW YORK

This book is designed to inform you of the nature, effects, and hazards of cocaine use and abuse. This book is not intended as a substitute for professional medical advice or health care. Neither the authors nor the publishers advocate the use of cocaine. The unprescribed use, possession, or sale of cocaine is illegal.

THE COKE BOOK: THE COMPLETE REFERENCE TO THE USES AND ABUSES OF COCAINE

A Berkley Book / published by arrangement with
Bookmark Books, Inc.

PRINTING HISTORY
Berkley edition / October 1984
Second printing / August 1986

For information address: The Berkley Publishing Group,
200 Madison Avenue, New York, New York 10016.

ISBN: 0-425-10021-9

A BERKLEY BOOK ® TM 757,375

PRINTED IN THE UNITED STATES OF AMERICA

Grateful acknowledgment is made to the following for permission to reprint or adapt previously published material:

Esquire Magazine for "The Cold-Cash Value of Cocaine," which appeared in an article by Howard Kohn, "Cocaine: You Can Bank On It," October 1983, © 1983 by Esquire Magazine.

New York Magazine for "The Bottom Line In New York," which appeared in an article by Nicholas Pileggi, "There's No Business Like Drug Business," December 13, 1982, © 1982 by Nicholas Pileggi.

The Journal of Psychedelic Drugs for "A Brief History of Cocaine," adapted from "A Medical Chronology of Cocaine" by Dr. George R. Gay in "You've Come a Long Way, Baby! Coke Time for the New American Lady of the Eighties," Vol. 13, No. 4, October-December 1981, © 1981 by The Journal of Psychedelic Drugs. Also, chart "Cocaine's Chemical Structure" adapted from above.

The Journal of Psychedelic Drugs for "Probability of Adverse Reactions Relationship to Cocaine Dose," adapted from "Cocaine" by Dr. David E. Smith and Dr. Donald R. Wesson. Vol. 10, No. 4, October-December 1978, © 1978 by The Journal of Psychedelic Drugs.

Dr. Mark S. Gold for *Behavioral and Physiological Effects Correlated with Neurotransmitters* from "Neuropsychopharmacology of Cocaine" by Dr. Mark S. Gold, Director of Research, Fair Oaks Hospital, Summit, N.J., © 1984 by Dr. Mark S. Gold.

The Food & Drug Book Co. Inc. for "Personal Cocaine Use Inventory," adapted from "Personal Drug Use Inventory" in THE LITTLE BLACK PILL BOOK, Lawrence D. Chilnick, ed., Bantam Books Inc., 1983, © 1983 by the Food & Drug Book Co. Inc.

Ice Nine Publishing Co. for lyrics excerpted from "Casey Jones" by The Grateful Dead, music by Jerry Garcia, words by Robert Hunter, © 1970 by Ice Nine Publishing Co.

ACKNOWLEDGMENTS

The staff of *The Coke Book* wishes to acknowledge the following special people whose time, help, professionalism, cooperation, and dedication have contributed to the value of this book:

Tom Holdorff, Nancy Sarnoff, photographic assistants.

Kenneth Youngstein, President—Biocom Ltd., for generous use of his facilities and personal support.

Rona Hunter for her professional and conceptual assistance in the creation of this book and the color insert.

Julie Seleman-Surrey, for word processing and production assistance.

Noel Silverman, James Miglino and Ned Leavitt, for their personal support and professional guidance.

Special thanks to Dr. Mark S. Gold, and his staff, including Barbara Capone, Linda Becker, Mary Beth Lincoln, and other personnel at Fair Oaks Hospital, Summit, N.J.

For their expertise and assistance, special thanks to Dr. Karl Verebey, Jamil Alrazi, Elizabeth Howard, Cindy Knoeller, and the staff of Psychiatric Diagnostic Laboratories of America Ltd.

Dr. George R. Gay, Dr. Donald R. Wesson, Millicent Buxton and the entire staff of the Haight-Ashbury Free Medical Clinic, whose assistance in this project and others has always been invaluable.

Ms. Gareth Esersky, our dedicated, persevering editor and her assistant, Sallye Leventhal.

Our gratitude to the many individuals whose personal stories and experiences have added to our knowledge and understanding of cocaine use and abuse, and a special thanks to Kaypro Computers.

FOREWORD

by David E. Smith, M.D.

Founder and Medical Director

Haight-Ashbury Free Medical Clinic
San Francisco

Through the 1960s and 1970s, due to many complicated, and interrelated, social and cultural factors, the reputation of cocaine was a drug neither widely abused nor dangerous. During those two decades, cocaine consumers, as well as some medical authorities, described the drug as a benign chemical that could not result in addiction, overdose, toxic psychosis, or death.

We seriously questioned such opinions.

Here in Haight-Ashbury, we witnessed the epidemic of amphetamine abuse during the late 1960s. Amphetamine, a central nervous system stimulant similar in action to cocaine, had, like cocaine, been touted as safe.

By the late 1970s our concerns about cocaine use proved to be well-founded, as we observed a significant increase in cocaine abuse, with parallel increases in cocaine overdose deaths, toxic consequences on physical, psychological and behavioral functioning, and the development of cocaine addiction characterized by compulsion, loss of control over the drug, and continued use despite adverse consequences.

By 1983, 19 percent of all first-time admissions at the Haight-Ashbury Free Medical Clinic's Outpatient Drug Detoxification Project were cocaine abusers, up 3 percent from 1980. This significant increase is, in part, the result of the clinic's specialized cocaine treatment programs, which accounted for approximately half of all drug treatment programs in San Francisco. But data on the city's overall drug treatment picture compiled between 1978 and 1982 by J. Newmeyer ("Drug Abuse Trends in the San Francisco Bay Area: June 1983," Report of the Haight-Ashbury Free Medical Clinic) confirm a similarly significant increase throughout San Francisco. While heroin and other opiates remain the major drugs of abuse (other than alcohol), cocaine is the source of the most rapidly developing problem.

During the five years beginning in 1978, the San Francisco Coroner reported a hike in cocaine overdose death rates *in excess of 300 percent*. Other major urban areas, such as Los Angeles, Denver and Miami, report similar increases in cocaine overdoses, and in patients seeking help for cocaine abuse. It is interesting to note that as cocaine moved out of the drug subculture into the mainstream of society, we saw a rise of cocaine abuse among younger physicians, a pattern first seen a century ago when cocaine use first became evident.

According to information available today, it is apparent that we are in the middle of a cocaine abuse epidemic in many major urban areas across the country. This produces a critical challenge for both our treatment system and society as a whole.

Approximately 75 percent of the new cocaine abusers swept up in this epidemic are employed. Their awareness of cocaine's hazards came to them only *after* they became users. As a group, they tend to be "treatment naive," which means they have not generally had repeated contact with the drug treatment system. Thus they are not "traditional" drug abusers or addicts aware of the availability of programs that might help them. While they seek help from a variety of sources, only some are appropriate.

Because of our treatment experience with close to 3,000 outpatient cocaine abusers, and our work with still more inpatient abusers, the Haight-Ashbury Free Medical Clinic can clearly define the major treatment considerations that should be a part of any worthwhile treatment program.

Cocaine withdrawal is not complicated by the kind of life-threatening seizures which require careful medication that are commonly experienced by those withdrawing from alcohol. But it does require supportive care which focuses on good nutrition, adequate sleep, and various procedures designed to help with insomnia due to anxiety.

It is also important, for both treatment specialists and cocaine abusers alike, to take note that cocaine may create a "kindling effect" through which cocaine abusers (and, for that matter, amphetamine abusers) who kick cocaine but return to the drug experience increasingly toxic reactions, at lower doses, with each relapse. With repeated withdrawals, each becomes more uncomfortable than the one before, and each return to cocaine produces more serious physical and emotional difficulties.

Family therapy can be extremely helpful to the cocaine abuser, and group therapy, where recovering cocaine abusers support one another in their efforts to resist the drug, can be critically important.

An exercise program helps make recovery a positive process, and actually reduces the urge for cocaine by changing the body's natural chemical balance (a process that occurs after twenty minutes or so of activity strenuous enough to stimulate the heart).

The recovering cocaine abuser must be convinced that any return to cocaine, even "just one more time," can be a serious relapse, since almost everybody who tries cocaine "just one more time" quickly returns to the previous pattern of abuse. For cocaine abusers, there is no such thing as "controlled use" or "cure." However, recovery—learning to live a comfortable and responsible life without the use of psychoactive drugs—is possible.

Much is known today about cocaine addiction, and ways to deal with it. *The Coke Book* is a significant step towards making available the most up-to-date knowledge about cocaine's history, its modern record of misuse and abuse, and its danger to individuals and society alike.

While researchers, physicians, and the general public continue to learn more about cocaine, there is without question a great deal that remains unclear or controversial. It is therefore important that those of us involved in drug abuse treatment keep searching for new techniques that might be helpful in showing cocaine abusers how they can lead full, productive lives without this dangerous drug.

CONTENTS

BOXES and CHART LIST

1
INTRODUCTION: A WORD TO THE WISE

There's nothin' like coke.

No other illicit drug ever burst so explosively onto the American scene.

Coke has had an economic impact on our country equal only to alcohol's.

The drug is responsible for an unprecedented nationwide increase in the rate of violent crime, especially murder.

It critically affects the way we look at our Hollywood stars, sports heroes, and even business executives.

Cocaine has spawned an entirely new type of drug abuser and drug dealer: the middle-class man or woman, from the early 30s to mid-40s in age, who has the same aspirations, hobbies, or habits as, and cannot be distinguished from, your own neighbor.

Cocaine's spread from coast to coast has changed the very definition of a drug addict. The old image of junkies in "Needle Park" no longer applies. Coke addicts can be the guy in the next office, wearing a three-piece suit . . . the young mother pushing her baby down the street . . . the welder on the assembly line.

But despite the new, obvious changes in the status of coke, cocaine abuse is not a new phenomenon. The drug has seen many previous peaks of popularity—though none the equal of today's—and has been in and out of fashion for more than a century.

FLOWER CHILDREN OF TODAY?

Yes, the '60s were filled with drugs—primarily pot, pills, and hallucinogens like LSD. But their impacts weren't the same.

Drug money in the '60s was nothing compared to today's cocaine fortunes. And the pot dealers—entrepreneurial flower children—certainly didn't resemble the ruthless daredevils who bring the "lady" to market today. However, many of yesterday's flower children are today's businessmen and professionals, "doing" coke as a matter of course. The previous permissive attitudes toward drugs paved the way to making cocaine socially acceptable today.

It is no coincidence that when Hollywood remade the classic gangster film *Scarface*, a vile cocaine boss was selected as the modern equivalent of the 1930s' rum-running gangster.

What changed? Why has the use of cocaine become so widespread this time around?

There are three reasons. First, cocaine today is readily available. And second, occasional use of the drug is relatively inexpensive.

Also, coke in recent years gained a new widespread "reputation" as a glamour drug. When illicit cocaine became the drug of stars in the late '70s, it also became a fashion and style influence which affected us all. By 1980, a veritable cocaine boom was well underway.

As early as 1980, tiny gold cocaine spoons and razor blades were *de rigueur* pieces of equipment among urban cowboys. The decor of one legendary

New York disco featured a giant moon with a coke spoon.

Altered, too, is the perception of cocaine held by science and medicine. What sages like Sigmund Freud only suspected, a century ago, has now been proven true: coke is a potent substance, a dangerous, addictive drug whose medical value is questionable.

DESTRUCTIVE FORCE

Cocaine's allure is still irresistible to many people, despite the fact that it all too often shows itself to be a destructive force in their lives.

This book shows how cocaine can influence all our lives today, even if we don't use it. *The Coke Book* explores our actual knowledge of the drug...how coke has spread through wide segments of our society...how it has created serious health problems for those who choose to use it...and how it threatens the safety of us all.

The problems result not only from the dangers of cocaine itself, but often from the adulterants used to cut cocaine. By the time it is sold on the street, adulterants may comprise the bulk of the purchase.

Most pot smokers can tell the difference between oregano and a smoke of good Marin County buds. But what a typical coke user buys for about $100 a gram can be almost anything, in any quantity and in unknown combinations. Even when the purchase *does* contain some real cocaine, it probably has several other ingredients as well.

Someone who pops tranquilizers knows the dosage he is taking—5 mg, 10 mg, etc. But cocaine users don't really know how much of that gram of "cocaine" they are about to ingest is really cocaine . . . how much of it is one or another of several possible adulterants or additives . . . or what the exact dosage of each adulterant is.

The addition of unknown quantities of often obscure chemicals, in fact, is one of the most overlooked aspects of cocaine use today.

This problem becomes a major issue when one considers that the adulterants might include heroin or a similarly dangerous drug, and that a good-time cocaine dosage for one person can be a deadly dosage for another. How can you be sure about the purity of your cocaine? This is one of many issues explored in this book, which includes a section of color photos of a simple test to determine the purity of a cocaine sample, and a complete description of the cocaine bleach test in Chapter 5.

ILLEGAL BUT AVAILABLE

Cocaine is an illegal drug under United States law. Its possession or sale carries stiff penalties.

But it is an accessible drug today, as easy to buy as any legal drug. The cocaine industry is responsible for a vast underground, and an enormous unregulated and untaxed economy. Few people realize just how extensive and virulent is the illicit cocaine trade.

Countless businesses in cities and towns across the United States have been started with cash stemming from cocaine. Condominiums and other high-rise buildings rest on foundations of illicit cocaine money. In some parts of the country, entire banking establishments are kept afloat by enormous infusions of illicit cocaine cash. And this underground cash has far-reaching economic consequences, not only for this country, but nations thousands of miles away. A full discussion of cocaine's economic impact can be found in Chapter 4.

The widespread use of cocaine by professionals in positions of responsibility—Wall Street brokers, airline pilots, corporate CEO's, and surgeons, to name just a few—has an impact on our lives not only in economic ways. It can become a matter of life and death for us. When the judgment of these professionals is impaired by cocaine, their perceptions of reality are altered, and their responses to critical situations are changed.

Entire businesses may fail. Or, worse, innocent people may be injured, even killed. This side of the cocaine story is detailed in Chapter 17.

Similarly, when the drug is used by society's heroes whose work we revere—athletes, rock stars, movie idols—it grants "doing" cocaine the status of acceptability, changing our way of looking at life, and altering our most fundamental values. Illicit cocaine is suddenly no longer reprehensible. The very people we, and our children, select as role models are doing it; it therefore becomes all right for us, too. For details, see Chapters 15 and 16.

Along with the breakdown of inhibitions about using this illicit drug, the social pressures grow to be "one of the crowd." *Everybody* does it, after all—the lawyer, the doctor, the accountant, our best friend. So why not?

COCAINE MISINFORMATION

People often don't know enough about cocaine to make an educated judgment about its use. One person using coke occasionally was told there was no certain scientific information about the drug's ability to cause exhilaration, or prolong the intensity of sexual intercourse. His reply: "Yeah, but it's fun."

Is it? There is no debate that millions of people use illicit cocaine for fun. Many *do* have a good time, without becoming addicts. Still, they often are not informed consumers. Unfortunately, people tend to approach cocaine with rather naive attitudes.

In an effort to downplay the drug's adverse effects, many cocaine users will say, "Well, it's a *natural* drug. It comes from a plant." Left unsaid is the assumption that because it comes from a plant, cocaine is harmless. Coke does start out as a shrub grown in the Andes mountains of South America (see Chapter 6), and the leaves of the coca plant are routinely chewed by the local peoples, with minimal, at least short-range, ill effects.

But by the time cocaine hits the streets of North America, it is far from a benign substance. Greatly refined, and with other substances mixed in, it can be deadly. The dose is unregulated . . . the precise composition of what is sold as cocaine is untested . . . and the environmental and other personal variables of the user can't be controlled.

The end result is that coke can be harmful in small doses, as well as large ones, depending on a host of factors which this book explores in Chapters 8–13.

There are people who choose cocaine as a recreational drug, and they owe it to themselves to know as much as possible about every one of the drug's potential effects and dangers. And they need to be aware of cocaine's psychologically addictive properties.

They should know how to recognize a side effect and a dangerous adverse reaction, just as they should be aware of a prescription drug's possible bad effects.

They should know the many cautions and warnings associated with cocaine use. For example, should cocaine be taken by a nursing mother? Someone who has a cold? One who suffers from high blood pressure? How do you know when you've had enough? Or when your reactions are not "normal"? Such information is not at the fingertips of most people when cocaine is passed around at a cocktail party. Yet, knowing about it may be critically important. It could be a matter of life and death.

THE COKE SUBCULTURE

Cocaine's discovery by the media has given it a whole new image. Coke is a "subject" for cover stories, movies, songs and books.

Cocaine now has its own subculture. There are networks of coke users, connected to networks of coke distributors. In fact, the effectiveness of the cocaine distribution system is one of the reasons for the drug's widespread use. Coke is something you can easily get your hands on. But unlike fads promoted by the media and then dropped, coke doesn't appear to be going away.

For an estimated 5,000 daily new coke users, and for the many millions of others who have already tried cocaine, the information contained in this book should become an essential part of their drug information.

Drug experts, as well as laymen, are increasingly worried about cocaine's power. One of the country's leading drug-abuse specialists, Dr. David E. Smith, founder and medical director of the Haight-Ashbury Free Medical Clinic in San Francisco, says that coke is a drug that's "so good, you shouldn't try it even once."

The California clinic's training director, Richard B. Seymour, agrees that cocaine's dangers are great. "It's hard to find anyone these days," he says, "who thinks coke has any redeeming factors."

"If cocaine would be legalized," says Dr. Mark Gold, director of research at both Fair Oaks Hospital, and New York City's Regent Hospital, and founder of the nationwide 800-COCAINE hotline, "based on the behavior observations, there would be a great increase in the numbers and severity of cocaine overdoses and toxicity."

The coke scene is neither simple to describe nor easy to study in a scientific manner. For example, the coke now being sold on the West Coast is very pure and also very inexpensive when compared to cocaine available today along the Atlantic seaboard, according to Dr. Seymour. Cocaine is notably cheaper than top-quality pot in California—about $70–90 a gram (compared to about $125 a gram in New York, where it is only 30–60 percent pure).

The cheap, high-quality drug is invading California, he says, because law enforcement officials have started shutting down the traditional smuggling havens of the Southeastern U.S. Thus the flow of cocaine in California shifts according to law enforcement priorities established in Florida and Texas, and is exceptionally difficult to accurately survey.

The Coke Book provides the most accurate, up-to-date information available on cocaine's use, the route it takes to the streets, homes and offices of America, and the drug's dangers.

The Coke Book is *not* a consumer's handbook, nor is it a "how-to" guide. It is, instead, a factual volume written for those who understand they need to know just what this white powder is, what it can do to those using it, and what it has already done to society. Is cocaine truly a "lady"? Or is it the out-of-control "white tornado" that free-basers talk about?

By carefully reading *The Coke Book,* you'll have all the information at hand, and you will be able to make your own judgment about cocaine.

2
COKE IN THE 1980s—POPULARITY AND PROBLEMS

Cocaine's psychoactive properties, together with the economics involved in coke's distribution and sale, make coke more popular today than any other black-market drug in America.

As it is bought and sold on the street, cocaine earns up to ten times more revenue than drugs like heroin. Because of widespread demand it is easier to sell than all the rest.

Even minuscule amounts of cocaine bring small-time traffickers an inordinately high return on their investments. The single shipment of a mere kilogram of cocaine from South America, brought into Florida by commercial airplane and handed over to a few distributors, might cost a small-time smuggler $15,000, including expenses like airplane tickets and hotel rooms.

It will sell just a few hours later for between $30,000 and $50,000—or more if the coke is of unusually good quality. It will eventually be worth about $100,000 when it is sold on the street in packets of a gram or less.

But cocaine enters the United States not just by the kilogram. Government officials estimate seventy-five *tons* of cocaine come into this country illegally every year, eventually costing the American economy as much as 40 *billion* dollars annually in lost productivity, sick days, expensive cocaine-caused accidents, thefts, and similar losses. And this figure does not include the billions of dollars spent on buying cocaine, which would otherwise probably be spent on more conventional goods and services.

So significant is the money generated by cocaine that government officials are worried about the very heart of America's economy—its banks. If bank deposits of cocaine money dry up, they fear, several of the smaller financial institutions around the United States would be in danger of collapse.

"COKE ECONOMY"

Businesses, too, rely on cocaine money for growth. Many firms, both large and small, were started (sometimes unwittingly) on cocaine capital, and some make liberal use of it for expansion. Elaborate money-washing schemes—quick transfers of funds from one account to another in overseas banks not subject to U.S. federal & state law—hide the origins of cocaine money prior to investment here (see Chapter 4).

Government investigators—even those not prone to hyperbole—say cocaine money, if taxed like other commodities, could provide the answer to the enormous national debt.

Cocaine is bought and sold on Wall Street . . . on the farm . . . on factory assembly lines . . . in the locker rooms of both professional and amateur athletes . . . in school corridors and classrooms . . . virtually everywhere people gather for work or recreation.

And this broad base of cocaine users, anxious for the "high" of a snort or a puff, keeps the industry growing stronger every week.

Over the past few years, cocaine has become a business so large it dwarfs the total value of some of America's most talked-about new national defense systems. Cocaine matches the automobile industry in economic power.

THE BOTTOM LINE IN NEW YORK

Amount of money generated by the illegal drug trade compared with major industries, in New York City.*

Illegal Drugs	$45,000,000,000
Retail Trade	$24,500,000,000
Garment Trade	$17,000,000,000
Manufacturing	$14,600,000,000
Tourism	$3,000,000,000
Entertainment	$2,500,000,000

Number of employees engaged in illegal drugs compared to those in major industries, in New York City.*

Wholesale and Retail Trades	595,000
Manufacturing	497,000
Illegal Drugs	100,000–300,000
Garment Trade	142,000
Construction	84,000

NOTE: Adapted with permission from an article by Nicholas Pileggi, "There's No Business Like Drug Business," NEW YORK Magazine, December 13, 1982, p. 40.

*According to the latest New York City figures.

THE COLD CASH VALUE* OF COCAINE

ROLLS-ROYCE (Silver Spirit)
775 grams = $93,000

MAJOR LEAGUE BASEBALL TEAM
166,667 grams = $20,000,000

BLOOMINGDALE'S MOST EXPENSIVE SUIT (a Giorgio Armani)
5 grams = $645

OCEANFRONT HOME IN THE BAHAMAS
10,000 grams = $1,200,000

VAN GOGH PAINTING
43,333 grams = $5,200,000

ROUND TRIP TO PARIS VIA CONCORDE
34 grams = $4,120

PRODUCTION OF A MAJOR MOVIE
106,250 grams = $12,750,000

NEW YACHT
1,666 grams = $200,000

THREE MOUNTINGS BY A PRIZEWINNING STALLION
3,333 grams = $400,000

NEW YORK RESTAURANT
4,767 grams = $500,000

NOTE: Adapted with permission from "Cocaine: You Can Bank On It," by Howard Kohn, ESQUIRE, October 1983, pp. 78–79.

*Based on current street value.

HOW DO YOU STOP A FLOOD?

Despite the size of the cocaine business, only about one out of every seven illegal shipments is intercepted by United States Customs officers.

The smugglers are too sophisticated and too numerous, say customs officials, for easy interception. Their weapons range from expensive handguns to elaborate automatic weapons suitable for commando raids to high-speed aircraft capable of avoiding America's most sophisticated radar defense networks. Such equipment far surpasses that available to drug enforcement agents.

From time to time, however, a cocaine seizure also nets some of these weapons, and perhaps even an airplane. Those are days of celebration for drug agents, since they are permitted to use the confiscated weapons—even the aircraft—in their war against cocaine. On April 24, 1984, officials seized an Eastern Airlines L-1011 jumbo jet, after a flight to Miami from Peru and Panama, when three pounds of cocaine were discovered hidden among electronic equipment. They returned the jet only after airline executives agreed to take several anti-smuggling steps.

Another factor affecting the official fight against cocaine is the social status of so many coke users.

For the most part, until a decade ago, cocaine had been used mainly by the very wealthy, a group relatively small in number but powerful in political influence. There was no notable government effort to crush the cocaine trade aimed at the well-to-do, important individuals. Or coke was thought to be used by musicians, artists, or blacks; it was never a drug of the middle class until the 1980s, when cocaine became the drug of choice among ever-increasing numbers of the upper middle class who were not likely to steal or commit other crimes to support their drug purchases.

And even though cocaine use is rapidly increasing among lower economic groups, it is not yet surrounded by the kind of public uproar that led to stern enforcement measures aimed at heroin.

To be sure, more and more crimes are committed to support cocaine habits across the country. In Florida—Miami in particular, where cocaine smugglers and distributors protect their territories and illicit industry—there has been a dramatic increase in the rate of drug-related murders.

There are varying estimates of the extent of current cocaine use. One expert asserts that 15,000,000 Americans use the drug on a regular basis, while another puts the figure closer to 25,000,000, with as many as twice that number having tried coke. And researchers predict that cocaine's spread won't peak for another half decade.

5,000 A DAY

Most agree that at least 5,000 individuals try coke for the first time, every day, and some experts say that fully 10 percent of all high school students have tried cocaine—or what they thought was cocaine. Recent studies show that cocaine use among young professionals in their 20s and 30s doubles each year.

As recently as fifteen years ago, surveys of drug use on college campuses classified cocaine with morphine and heroin in a single question. In one study of 517 people, not a single student reported having used cocaine more than a few times.

But by 1978, nearly a third of the students surveyed said they used cocaine regularly. What makes this even more significant is that morphine and heroin use hadn't changed at all. On college campuses today, coke consumption ranks second only to marijuana use.

ADVERTISING COKE

Since the mid-1970s, cocaine use has been promoted primarily by word of mouth, a technique which any Madison Avenue executive will agree is the most effective form of advertising to any segment of the population, whether white-collar or blue-collar worker, ghetto dweller or Hollywood star.

It is ironic that until recently even extensive negative publicity about cocaine—its health hazards, high costs, impurities, etc.—seemed only to make it more appealing.

It is possible that one of coke's most appealing qualities is its "famous"—or "infamous"—status. "Famous" people (and everyone wants to be famous like movie stars and rock musicians) have been known to use this drug. Indeed, cocaine has a reputation for providing the best "high" available.

Studies that show coke's debilitating power are now counteracting the "famous" image. Two studies, one at UCLA and another conducted in the nation's capital, show cocaine's enormous power. In these studies, apes and monkeys were offered unlimited quantities of cocaine. In both cases, the subjects preferred the cocaine to food, sex, or any other drug. (See Chapter 13.)

UCLA's Ron Siegel, a well-known pharmacologist and cocaine expert, calls cocaine "*the* most rewarding and reinforcing drug for a primate . . . whether he has a tail or a $100,000 income. Primates like cocaine!"

BUYERS AND SELLERS

Those who can afford to buy cocaine on a regular, perhaps daily, basis are for the most part affluent.

But many of those who *sell* cocaine are chronic users who can't afford the drug except as a profit from their sales. They often sell the worst coke, "cut" many times with a variety of other chemicals to increase the profit margin, which usually means a few more grams of cocaine for themselves.

One's degree of access to cocaine tends to control its effect and use. Those with high incomes, who can afford more coke—and pay for the highest quality—find themselves addicted because they can afford to be. Other, poorer users may avoid addiction until the price comes down; their access increases through dealing, or they turn to crime for added cash.

HOW COCAINE IS USED

One way to understand cocaine use is to see *how* the drug is used. There are five "levels" of cocaine use recognized by the National Commission of Marijuana and Drug Abuse:

EXPERIMENTAL: Short-term, irregular "trial" usage, either by snorting or smoking free-base. Experimental users are primarily motivated by curiosity and a desire to experience such drug effects as euphoria and a presumed enhancement of sexual performance. Experimental use usually ends either after the curiosity is satisfied, or, when adequate supplies at a sufficiently low price become available to buy more cocaine, the use becomes regular.

SOCIAL USE: Commonly takes place among close groups of friends who wish to share an experience perceived as acceptable and pleasurable. As with experimental usage, social cocaine use is voluntary, and participants are usually only after some fun.

CIRCUMSTANTIAL/SITUATIONAL: Generally directed toward a specific task, for which cocaine is seen as a temporary "helper." Such usage is commonly self-limiting; once the particular effect is achieved, or the one-time need is met, cocaine is no longer used. Attempting to overcome a period of depression through cocaine would be one example of circumstantial or situational usage, as would coping with an especially rough task at the work place.

INTENSIFIED USE: Seen mostly among those who smoke cocaine free-base at least once a day. Generally these users believe they must use cocaine to maintain a certain level of performance, so they use the drug almost continuously for as much as five hours a day, one to two months at a time. These episodes of near-constant cocaine use are known as "runs."

COMPULSIVE USE: Characterized by high-frequency, high-intensity levels of cocaine use for exceptionally long periods, perhaps years. Compulsive use is inevitably followed by psychological and physical dependence, and a reduced ability to function socially. One of the main motivations of compulsive users is their desire to avoid withdrawal symptoms such as severe depression.

These patterns are closely linked to a user's occupation and economic status. While a social user may spend $100 a month on cocaine, and maintain a near normal life-style, the intensified user might spend up to $1,000 daily.

Compulsive, addicted users have been known to spend upwards of $12,000 a week! Such extravagant cocaine use almost always involves dealing in large amounts of coke, or engaging in some other criminal activity, although some "big-league" users are merely independently wealthy.

WHERE COKE IS USED

For Recreation: Cocaine is most often used in recreational settings, where "fun" is the focus. This accounts for its spread to many different classes of users. What group, after all, doesn't want to have fun? Cocaine's reputation as a glamorous drug—an enhancer of music, an aphrodisiac, an "energizer"—makes it an attractive choice to someone out for a good time.

To Enhance Performance: Cocaine's professed ability to ward off fatigue and enhance concentration makes it the "ideal" drug for those involved in repetitive tasks requiring that they stay awake for long periods of time while continuing to pay close attention to their work. Athletes believe that using coke helps them ignore the pain from violent contact sports and keeps them alert on the playing field, but it is an exaggerated sense of being in control which they probably experience. Coke use in this case is rarely just "circumstantial" but, rather, "chronic."

On the Job: Cocaine use often spreads among colleagues, either in the same profession or within groups of associates on the same economic or social level. People in many roles—athletes, physicians, salespeople, assembly-line workers, Wall Street brokers—use coke to change their perceptions of working conditions.

Coke is used on the job most frequently in the belief that it enhances performance. According to Dr. Joseph Pursch, Corporate Medical Director for the California-based Care Unit Hospitals—which treats some 40,000 drug and alchohol abusers each year—cocaine's psychologically addicting powers are those very properties of the drug which people rely on to help them at work. While physical addiction causes some withdrawal symptoms, and is certainly difficult to overcome, psychological addiction is much harder to kick. "A cocaine user feels that he can no longer dance or party," says Dr. Pursch, "or see his lover, without using cocaine."

"WHITE LINES ON THE JOB"

This book explores separately the extensive use of cocaine among the Hollywood set, throughout the sports world, and in the financial community (see Chapters 15, 16, and 17). In brief:

Wall Street: Cocaine appears to be the most sought-after drug in the country's financial community, where brokers and traders dealing with countless millions of dollars of other people's money are under constant stress, and where some require a continual chemical reminder that they can handle the jobs.

Athletics: Another group whose cocaine use is renowned includes men (and an increasingly large number of women) whose names are heard nearly every day on radio and TV, and are printed in the sports pages of newspapers. Athletes receive more publicity about cocaine abuse than almost any other segment of the work force. They are, after all, our heroes, and examples to our children.

But, like anyone else, they face pressures at work and in their personal lives. And, from time to time, athletes seek a little lift. Cocaine is frequently their drug of choice, since for many athletes the high cost of coke is no barrier. Additionally, cocaine is often given free to famous athletes by hangers-on who use the drug and who wish to ingratiate themselves with team members.

Other Professionals: Imagine yourself in a jumbo jet with 350 other passengers, flying over the Atlantic at 35,000 feet. The intercom system clicks and buzzes, but instead of a "Fasten Your Seat Belt" announcement, you overhear the navigator saying, "Hey, skipper, you gotta introduce me to the man supplyin' your coke. That stuff last night was stu-*pen*-dous!"

Scary? Certainly. Yet increasingly, commercial airline pilots—as well as architects, engineers, lawyers, and other professionals—are using cocaine because they believe it boosts their alertness and improves their performance in the cockpit, in court, or at the drafting table where critical decisions are made about whether a new building will stand up under its own weight.

Most—but not all—professionals who find themselves in trouble with drugs get treatment, often sponsored by their bosses. Large corporations have found it much less expensive to treat drug abuse than replace the employee. Others, like prominent Manhattan attorney James Tannian, get indicted instead. The lawyer faces charges of stealing $275,000 from the estate of a wealthy widow to support his expensive cocaine habit.

Even Congressmen are not immune. California Democrat John Burton admits he spent $100,000 on cocaine while representing San Francisco's Golden Gate district in Washington. Several anti-drug laws were passed during Burton's tenure in the Capitol, and he insists he was a "very effective" representative despite his coke addiction.

Medicine: Among physicians, drug addiction is estimated to be many times the rate of the rest of society, basically because drugs are so plentiful, and stress is so inherent in a physician's life-style. About one percent of all doctors become drug-dependent at some point in their professional lives. Nurses and other medical workers have drug-abuse rates almost as high as doctors, according to national statistics.

The American Medical Association, like other professional medical groups, understandably downplays such alarming statistics in order to maintain the stature of member physicians. Many addicted doctors remain in practice, "carried" by colleagues who understand that discovery means loss of license and livelihood.

Recently, however, the AMA began a series of regional programs for so-called "impaired physicians." Participants remain at work after joining the program, despite the development of symptoms typical of the addicted: deterioration of personal health, loss of interest in work, and emotional disorders.

It is not too farfetched today to picture a surgeon, anesthesiologist, or other medical professional "unwinding" after a hard day's work with a few milligrams of cocaine, and wondering—worrying—whether a colleague will learn of the indiscretion. It is only a small step further to imagine that same physician scrubbing up for surgery only minutes after the last "hit." It's a common plot for television, but a very real situation.

Cocaine is only one of the countless drugs readily available to medical workers, and it remains far behind prescription-controlled narcotics as a primary drug of abuse. But hundreds of physicians around the country have used cocaine extensively, and its use, say experts, appears to be growing.

HOW CAN YOU TELL?

Businesses have begun dealing more realistically with professionals, executives and laborers who abuse cocaine in order to keep going on the job.

One of the significant problems on-the-job cocaine abuse presents is that it's exceptionally difficult to detect. Determining when an executive is high on coke, or when the same individual is simply over-enthusiastic about the latest contract, is much harder than detecting an assembly-line worker whose output suddenly doubles.

Often, cocaine abuse among executives occurs during luncheons or dinner meetings, and is easily overlooked. The very nature of executive work—continuous decision-making, a constant rush to complete tasks—often lets executives continue performing while on drugs. Coke promises a "boost" to these business leaders if they can refrain from using it excessively. Only after a long period of serious abuse are they likely to be discovered by superiors as cocaine users.

An assembly-line welder, on the other hand, is more quickly discovered when his work becomes either incompetent or obviously performed in haste. While a short-term use of the drug will probably go unnoticed, and may even improve the worker's productivity and apparent high interest in the job, even moderate use is likely to be quickly uncovered due to decline in work performance.

Attitudes towards drug abuse on the job vary depending on the specific drug involved. For example, heroin use is almost universally abhorred in the work place, yet popping tranquilizers can show that "you are in a high-powered job, filled with stress," explains one employment counselor, and therefore taking advantage of a recognized remedy.

In some industries, cocaine use is viewed as an acceptable response to the demands of the job. However, cocaine abuse at work frequently involves dealing in the drug across job lines; that is, a manager buys coke from a subordinate; a foreman sells to a laborer. Thus, abuse on the job is often covered up until it's too late.

More and more, companies are attempting to uncover drug abuse even before an employee is hired, by screening job applicants—executives and laborers alike—for drug use before putting them on the payroll. The results of pre-employment urine and blood tests have astounded business leaders. One prominent West Coast chemical company reports that fully half of all job applicants being tested for current drug use showed positive results on medical tests, and in subsequent interviews, only a small handful tried to deny their involvement with drugs such as cocaine.

Companies are also beginning to discover that the corporate approach to cocaine abuse can deeply affect employee morale. Workers are aware of who, in their ranks, is having trouble with drugs, and they keep a close watch on the firm's actions.

According to Dr. Mark Gold, if co-workers see a cocaine user returning from treatment looking and feeling better, and witness the company's willingness to consider the former drug abuser an unwitting victim rather than a destructive influence, the co-workers will be inclined to devote more energies to their work.

Corporations, however, tend to treat drug abuse with more confidentiality than sports teams. While companies will often send their executives on vacation, professional sports team members are more often suspended, and usually publicly chastised and humiliated.

Many companies have established Employee Assistance Programs (EAPs), and use in-house ombudsmen or specialists, to deal with individual cases of drug abuse.

Numerous professional sports organizations are beginning to approach the problem in an even more businesslike manner, for good reason: they are both businesses and teams. They are attempting to reduce the publicity surrounding individual cases of cocaine abuse, and trying to draw cocaine users into treatment programs. A summary of professional sports organizations' stands on cocaine will be found in Chapter 16.

The National Football League, along with other professional sports organizations, has in recent years become much tougher in its handling of drug-abusing players. "NFL players occupy a unique position in the eyes of the public," says Commissioner Pete Rozelle.

"They are the objects of admiration and emulation by young people. Involvement with illegal drugs poses numerous risks to the integrity of professional football and the public's confidence in it. Thus, every player must adhere to certain standards of personal conduct both on the field and off. Every player agrees by his employment contract not to engage in activities detrimental to the sport."

The NFL, Rozelle points out, must often act in ways different from law enforcement agencies, suspending players even though they haven't been prosecuted. While the league will guarantee treatment for all players seeking it, this policy is "not intended to relieve all players of personal responsibility for illegal drug involvement."

The league tries to address this problem on two fronts, according to Dan Rooney, president of the Pittsburgh Steelers. The first deals with education, the second with rehabilitation.

"Players who voluntarily report their problem to the clubs prior to any criminal involvement," he reports, "pursue treatment, and thereafter remain drug free, are not subject to league disciplinary action.

"NFL discipline is reserved for cases in which there is no dependency problem, or in which the player has concealed his problem and as a result has become entangled in the criminal justice system."

Similar policies are in force in the National Basketball Assn. and Major League Baseball. The NBA, however, can suspend players for life if they fail at a drug treatment program and return to drug use.

Until recently, baseball players, were less known for their cocaine use but were notorious for their alcohol problems. Some of this difference is due to the sociological background of the players, and some stems from the nature of the game.

Cocaine use among professional athletes—who are generally between eighteen and forty years old and "upscale"—is a natural, says Dr. Joseph Pursch. "Young, impressionable men who've grown up in small towns suddenly have big-city apartments, sophisticated girl friends, hot cars and spending money," he says.

On-the-job coke takes its toll on those who don't use it, too. Coaches report that they've returned to the college ranks from professional teams because they can't control drug use among the "adult" pros. One expert who treats players reports that several coaches have told him they simply can't work with "stoned" players.

"That's one of the reasons you see coaches who seem to be successful quitting and going back to colleges," he said.

THE PROBLEM THAT WON'T GO AWAY

Often, managers are reluctant to confront an obvious drug user despite the clear symptoms. In these cases, only when offices are completely disrupted does intervention occur.

Several executives report "waiting months too long," before addressing the problem of a drug user. One corporate leader said he finally fired a worker because the employee had become inefficient and unreliable, but the executive added: "I never considered drugs as the problem until after he had been fired and another employee told me.

"Two things struck me as odd," the businessman continued. "First, why didn't I pick up on it. And second, why didn't anyone in the office mention it to me.

"I think the main reasons were my attitude and our policy. There is no strong, stated policy. We ran the kind of organization where ultimate performance was important and each employee has a lot of leeway.

"Thus, without any clear-cut rules, each person does his own thing. I think both the company and the employee were badly served by the lack of stated policy or rules. It was clearly a serious mistake. This was a valuable and loyal employee. It broke my heart to have to let him go."

This wait-and-see attitude is one of the reasons addiction and abuse become widespread in businesses and sports organizations. Until recently, the policies of professional sports teams have been to deal with players only after they've reached the point of dysfunction, or turned themselves in.

But now teams have begun to consider changing policies that would bring them into line with some other industries. Public service organizations—nuclear reactor workers are an example—are now requiring weekly drug screens.

Unfortunately, there is a lack of consistency in rules among industries. Military pilots must be "drug free," for example, but commercial pilots are not regularly screened for drug use (although efforts are underway to require regular drug testing).

Strong union rules often prevent management from acting when drug use is suspected, until someone runs into trouble with the law. This is especially evident in the sports world. Player associations have protected their members and, in general, an adversary relationship with management exists in professional sports. But professional sports are changing, too—out of necessity.

Professional sports organizations, which are trying to avoid lawsuits by season ticket holders (and even other players) angered by drug-caused poor team performance, are beginning to write new regulations forcing more frequent drug tests, and requiring treatment when abuse is discovered. So obvious has the drug problem become that some players are, literally, carried off the field because they are "stoned" or "high."

3
USING COCAINE TODAY

Cocaine has an effect on the body regardless of how it enters the bloodstream and works its way to the brain. But the speed with which it takes effect, and the intensity of the drug's euphoric action, are determined by the method of use, the social setting, and the purity of the drug.

There are several common ways of using coke:

- Snorting cocaine powder,
- Smoking cocaine paste,
- Smoking cocaine free-base,
- "Chasing the dragon,"
- Injecting cocaine,
- Applying cocaine to the genitals.

Although coca leaves are chewed as a way of life in the Andes, drug experts here consider this form of use rather unlikely in the United States. As one expert says, "No one has ever come into an emergency room here with a coca leaf hanging out of his mouth."

Sometimes cocaine is used in combination with other drugs, such as heroin, amphetamine, marijuana, or a variety of other "uppers" or "downers." Such combinations are further discussed in Chapter 15.

DRUG CEREMONIES

Most drug use involves some kind of ritual. The most elaborate ceremonies, of course, surround alcohol, a drug which has gained nearly worldwide acceptance despite its addictive properties and its immeasurable costs to society, including millions of alcohol-related deaths, countless destroyed families, and a stunning loss to the economies of nations where alcoholism is rampant.

The United States, and most other countries, have nevertheless accepted alcohol as a quasi-official national drug. In Japan, the public drunkenness of businessmen on weekends has led to a cottage industry of mini–hotel rooms geared specifically to drying them out before the next workweek. Alcohol is blamed for much of Russia's economic weakness, yet even Moscow's rigid officials have never tried to completely stem the flow of vodka.

America's bout with prohibition is, of course, history, but repeal pointed out the national acceptance of a clearly dangerous drug, alcohol.

With acceptance of alcohol comes acceptance of the rituals surrounding its use. Drinking alcohol—wine, beer and hard liquor alike—is replete with ceremony. New Year's Eve champagne toasts . . . the sniffing and close inspection of a fine wine . . . the polite offer of pre-dinner drinks in homes from coast to coast . . . the casual passing of beer cans at a picnic, portrayed nightly in television commercials . . . all add to the eventual enjoyment of the drug itself.

Cocaine, too, even though its use is illegal, is surrounded by elaborate ceremony. Some studies even indicate that for occasional users of small doses, the ceremony is equal in importance to the drug itself. Researchers reporting in the prestigious publication *Scientific American* say that a group of "experienced cocaine users" was unable to tell the difference between cocaine and the local anesthetic lidocaine when sniffed through the nose.

Another study, conducted by the University of Chicago School of Medicine, indicated that when injected, cocaine could not be immediately distinguished from amphetamine, although cocaine's effects were more evident after several minutes.

The effects of cocaine, and other drugs which influence the mind, indeed "differ according to the expectations of the user, the setting or circumstances in which the drug is taken and the history and personality of the user," says one extensive research study.

Even the illegality of cocaine, which offers the possibility of arrest, is said to enhance the "high" for those who enjoy taking risks, much the same way the potential for serious injury or death accompanying such sports as sky-diving or hang-gliding is said to lure many individuals. A similar sense of adventure prevailed during Prohibition, when countless men and women were drawn as much to the excitement of the illegal speakeasy as to the drinks available only there.

Of course, using cocaine does not *require* an accompanying ritual. Many users snort, inject or free-base cocaine in the privacy of their homes or offices, just as drinkers enjoy a shot of bourbon or a bottle of beer at home. But today's cocaine experience is inextricably tied, for better or worse, to ceremony.

SNORTING COKE

Most social cocaine use involves "snorting," that is, inhaling the drug through the nose. The coke most often used for nasal inhalation has been processed in South America to a cocaine purity of about 82 percent. A rough *base* cocaine is dissolved in ether and mixed with hydrochloric acid. After the mixture is filtered and dried, fine crystals of cocaine hydrochloride remain. More than 100 pounds of cocaine HCl may be produced in a mere 15 minutes at each "crystal lab" where this work is done. Of course, these high-purity crystals—with the consistency of a fine powder—will be "cut" substantially with other ingredients by the time they reach a party in the U.S.

At parties and other functions where cocaine is made available, the presentation of the drug and the equipment used for snorting it represent the event's status as much as the table setting in a restaurant provides a strong clue to the restaurant's price range and the chef's abilities.

It is "essential," for example, for a host to present the cocaine on a spotlessly clean glass or polished marble surface, to be sure no guest is kept waiting more than a few moments, and to guarantee that the drug be of sufficient potency that even experienced users will notice the care taken in its purchase.

Some guests will provide their own coke and may offer it to others. But in high-income social circles, it is often considered impolite to accept more than a small sample; one is expected to use the cocaine provided by the host, or bring along one's own supply.

Elegant glass straws for drawing the drug into the nose are usually furnished, together with tiny "coke spoons" which some users prefer. A tightly-rolled dollar bill is frequently substituted for the straw, and some prefer using a $100 bill as an outward sign of wealth and status. While pre-rolled dollar bills may be offered by the host, higher denominations—according to the social etiquette of cocaine—should be provided by the guests.

Appropriate drinks are served to accompany the cocaine, most often rum or fine brandy.

The Presentation

On the flat glass or marble surface, the cocaine is finely chopped with a single-edged razor blade. Enormous profits have been earned by dealers in drug paraphernalia, who sell chopping kits for much more than their manufactured value. The kits might contain only a small mirror, a razor blade, and a few straws, but may retail for upwards of $15. More luxurious kits are bought for hundreds of dollars; their contents might have cost the supplier $20–30.

Several "lines" of the chopped cocaine are formed on the clean surface with deft manipulations of the razor blade. Each line is about two inches long and an eighth of an inch wide, roughly the size of the kind of string used for wrapping a parcel for mailing.

From a single gram of cocaine—the normal street purchase—about thirty lines can be made, each line containing somewhere between 25 and 35 milligrams of powder. The actual amount of cocaine present in each line depends on the purity of the drug.

As a tray of cocaine is passed around, each guest inhales a line through a straw into the nose.

The euphoria of one cocaine line lasts about twenty to thirty minutes. Most users will snort a second line when the first begins to wear off, and continue snorting until the supply of cocaine is depleted. A sign of a successful cocaine party is its duration; if the supply dwindles too early, then not enough cocaine was made available, and the party was only mediocre. The most "successful" cocaine parties last all night!

Because cocaine is a topical anesthetic, it numbs whatever body tissue it contacts. The numbing sensation which occurs during coke snorting is as much a part of the ritual as is chopping, drawing out the lines, and using the appropriate straw.

As cocaine crystals enter the nose, they dissolve on the moist walls of the mucous membranes and are absorbed by the many tiny blood vessels near the surface. Blood quickly carries molecules of coke to the brain.

Following cocaine snorting, the nose usually becomes congested. Symptoms similar to a head cold quickly develop, including sneezing and stuffiness. Any undissolved grains of cocaine remaining in the nose are likely to cause burning and soreness.

Some users employ a salt water mixture to flush out the inside of the nose after a round of snorting. Decongestant nose drops are also commonly employed to help keep the nose clear, and antihistamines—both over-the-counter and prescription—are used as well.

If cocaine is snorted frequently without adequate nasal cleaning, the cocaine residue can eventually dissolve the delicate membrane—and even cartilage—inside the nose, causing ulceration of the nasal septum, the tissue separating one nostril from the other.

Eventually, an actual hole may develop in the septum. This can be repaired only with surgery, after which even a minimal amount of cocaine can do *permanent* damage to the nose.

During the late '70s, a perforated septum was considered a status symbol among cocaine users, since it was evidence either of the financial ability to buy large amounts of the drug, or gain invitations to all the "right" parties where coke was served. Now, it is seen as a sign that the user was not cautious in handling the drug, or had unwisely overindulged to the point of ignoring proper safeguards.

SMOKING COCAINE PASTE

Cocaine smoking is almost never an individual's initiation into the drug's use. Most coke beginners start out by snorting the drug. But once they grow accustomed to the euphoria provided that way, many seek other, more intense, experiences with cocaine.

Smoking provides it.

Cocaine is smoked in two forms: as a paste, and as free-base.

Smoking cocaine paste first came to light in the United States about 1974. Reports of paste smoking originated in Peru, and then spread to other South American countries including Colombia, Bolivia, and Ecuador.

Coca paste is the first by-product of coca leaves after harvest. The leaves are crushed, then soaked in alcohol, mixed with benzol, and vigorously shaken. The alcohol is drained away, and sulfuric acid is added, followed by another shaking. Sodium carbonate is then added, and the result is a compound containing all the alkaloids—including cocaine—present in the leaf.

The compound is washed in kerosene or gasoline and cooled in a refrigerator to produce crude cocaine crystals with many impurities.

In Spanish, the end result is called *base* (pronounced "bah-say"), but is not the same as the extremely pure "free-base" product (described below), despite the similarity in names.

Another process for producing this raw cocaine compound is to dissolve the leaves in sulfuric acid, and mix in some sodium carbonate. This creates a gray-white or dull brown powder with a slightly sweet smell, which reminds some people of the scent of tobacco leaves.

Both methods result in an extremely potent substance which may be between 40 and 80 percent pure cocaine sulfate.

Other methods of extracting cocaine from coca leaves to form a very rough paste include one process in which powdered leaves are cooked with kerosene and baking soda, and another in which leaves are left to rot in water, then mixed with sulfuric acid to draw out the desired chemicals.

Throughout South America, coca paste is quite inexpensive compared to pure cocaine. The equivalent of a few dollars can provide days of exhilaration for a small group of Bolivian farmers, say, who have grown disenchanted with the mild experience provided by chewing raw coca leaves. In that continent, smoking coca paste frequently represents an individual's first significant use of any hard drug.

The dried paste is sometimes sprinkled on a marijuana cigarette for smoking, even though it still contains such undesirable substances as benzoic and sulfuric acids, methanol, several alkaloids other than cocaine, and residual kerosene.

More often, a tobacco cigarette is emptied, and the coca paste is inserted into the paper tube in alternate layers with the tobacco.

It is rare in the U.S. for anyone other than major suppliers to smoke cocaine paste, since here it is seldom sold in small quantities. Smugglers earn much more by further refining the paste before selling it.

Addiction to cocaine paste is common among its users. The "high" from inhaling paste smoke is about the same as taking coke by injection. It provides an extremely fast euphoria, which quickly fades, leading to severe depression unless the experience is repeated regularly. Psychotic reactions, as well as social and physical deterioration (weight loss, etc.) often accompany paste smoking. Furthermore this method leads to distortions of perception, dangerous changes in metabolism, and severe emotional problems. All of these are difficult to reverse.

SMOKING FREE-BASE

Free-base smoking is the most popular new form of recreational cocaine use in the United States. Although it resembles coca paste smoking, it is a substantially different activity, and has produced a large paraphernalia industry: many users buy a prepackaged "kit" to engage in this extremely dangerous form of coke use.

Cocaine free-base is just what its name implies—the cocaine base, free of adulterants, for smoking in its pure form. Free-base is created not from coca paste or *base*, but by dissolving the street cocaine—rarely more than 50 percent pure—in water, and using chemicals to extract the real stuff.

The highly flammable chemicals used in this process cause the drug-related fires and explosions we read about, such as the fire involving comedian Richard Pryor (see Chapter 15).

The introduction of free-basing in the United States probably took place by accident. Researchers looking into the subject say cocaine enthusiasts visiting South America misunderstood the meaning of *base,* and upon their return sought chemists who could make a pure "base" of cocaine from the impure drug bought on the streets.

According to the *Journal of Psychoactive Drugs*: "Thinking that *base* was simply cocaine free-base, they smoked according to the patterns they had observed in South America. These users were smoking a form of cocaine heretofore unknown among traditional patterns of use. The cocaine free-base differs from coca paste or crude cocaine *base* in that free-base does not contain companion cocaine alkaloids, solvents or other residue from the leaf extraction process."

The chemistry involved in making free-base cocaine is unusually simple. Cocaine hydrochloride, the active substance in street coke, can be extracted in a matter of minutes with basic equipment costing less than ten dollars.

Five methods are in common use today. Those which utilize flammable chemicals, such as ether, pose the great danger of causing explosions or serious fires because flames are also used to both make and smoke free-base.

1. *The "California Clean-up Method":* Street cocaine is dissolved in water, then treated with a base such as ammonia, and ether. The ether is separated and dried, leaving cocaine free-base crystals.

2. *The "Careful California Method":* Similar to the "Clean-up" method, but with careful controls of temperature and acidity. The crystals are washed with water, filtered, and more carefully dried.

3. *The "Baking-Soda Method"*: The street cocaine is boiled in water with baking soda, and the free-base is filtered out and dried.

4. *The "Ammonia Method"*: Ammonium hydroxide is mixed with the street cocaine, and the pure cocaine is filtered out of the mixture.

5. *The "Spoon Method"*: Street cocaine is mixed with water and ammonium hydroxide in a spoon, which is heated over a flame.

After Extraction

Once the free-base has been extracted, the cocaine is smoked in a water pipe. The purified molecules are carried straight to the brain in a few seconds.

Some free-basers make their own water pipes out of glass flasks, funnels, and a rubber stopper, but most buy commercially available equipment containing fine stainless steel screens that keep to a minimum the amount of cocaine lost during burning.

A small amount of the free-base cocaine is placed on the screen and lit with a match, lighter, or small bunsen-burner type torch.

The smoke passes through the liquid inside the water pipe before being inhaled, and the pipe is most often filled with rum, which afficionados insist gives a unique taste to the coke.

"Deep inhalation techniques, similar to those used with marijuana smoking, are employed," reports the *Journal of Psychoactive Drugs*. "Since the heat of combustion is so high, the screen remains hot for a period of time and users must wait for it to cool so as to prevent additional cocaine free-base from melting immediately. When several smokers are sharing a pipe, however, a larger amount of cocaine free-base is initially placed on the screen and the pipe is passed quickly from user to user so that the delay in gratification derived from smoking is minimal."

When smoking socially, the publication continues, "care is taken to apply a minimum of heat to the free-base and thus prevent it from flaming and producing a 'bad carbon taste.'"

The elaborate rituals surrounding social free-basing include filling balloons with exhaled smoke, which can be inhaled again later. Some users "will scrape the glass stems of the pipes, as well as the screens, in order to remove smokable materials," says the *Journal,* adding: "Still others claim the 'best' cocaine free-base is that which is re-obtained from the water in the pipe." According to the *Journal,* one user even said he smoked a supply of his own saliva, which contained some cocaine.

Lost in the Smoke

Laboratory studies demonstrate that smoking cocaine free-base in a water pipe gives the user significantly more exhilaration than cocaine free-base smoked as a cigarette. In addition, water-pipe smoking is less irritating to the mouth and throat, users report.

Close to half the psychoactive cocaine smoke drifts away from a cigarette's burning end, studies show, with only about 6 percent of the available cocaine actually entering the lungs. Even in a simple water pipe, not much more cocaine becomes available for smoking. But in a water pipe with adequate screens, and used with appropriate temperatures, substantially more cocaine can be inhaled. Furthermore, a top-quality water pipe will permit the recovery of much unburned cocaine through scraping and cleaning.

Smoking free-base cocaine causes a sudden, intense rush, accompanied by dilated pupils, a rapid heart rate, increased blood pressure, and fast breathing.

Feelings of energy, power, and competence are common. The euphoric high eventually subsides into a restless irritability, which sometimes causes the user to turn to heroin to relieve the tense and overstrung feeling. Sleep is impossible during a free-base binge.

Substantial weight loss is typical among free-base smokers. There also are reports of paranoid and psychotic reactions. Most free-base deaths, however, result from accidental fires rather than overdose. Still, sudden heart and respiratory failure leading to death has occurred among chronic users.

Individual tolerance to cocaine smoking depends on several factors (discussed in detail in Chapter 8), but in general, dependence and addiction occur rapidly. What starts out as a recreational or situational experiment often becomes an uncontrollable compulsion.

"CHASING THE DRAGON"

Another method of inhaling cocaine free-base smoke, while not exactly "smoking" it, is the increasingly popular technique called "dragon chasing."

The cocaine is placed on a sheet of aluminum foil and held over a small flame. As it melts, and tiny whisps of smoke rise from the puddle of cocaine, the smoke is inhaled deeply. The flame and foil can be easily manipulated to prolong the experience, said to be similar to water-pipe free-basing.

This is called "dragon chasing" or "chasing the dragon" because the smoke sometimes looks like a miniature dragon chasing its own tail. Originally used only with heroin in this country, it is a method common among opium smokers in the Far East, and is gaining rapid acceptance here for cocaine. Some cocaine free-basers prefer a water pipe for their cocaine, and "chase the dragon" with heroin to diminish the agitation caused by coke.

SHOOTING COKE

Injecting cocaine is viewed by many experts—both coke enthusiasts and physicians specializing in drug abuse—as akin to attempting suicide. Yet a tiny minority of cocaine users, approximately one percent, persists in using this exceptionally dangerous method.

The highs from intravenous coke are strong, but exceptionally brief. Since cocaine sold on the street is seldom intended for injections, it may contain impurities that can permanently damage the blood system, or prove fatal even in small doses. If a pure cocaine can be found for injection, it is prepared like heroin, and shooting galleries with candles, spoons, and used syringes are not uncommon sights around the country.

Ailments associated with shooting up on heroin—skin abscesses and hepatitis—frequently follow intravenous cocaine use as well. And the threat of overdose is substantially greater than with snorting coke, and somewhat greater than with smoking either cocaine paste or free-base.

It is hard to imagine why anyone would decide to inject cocaine, considering the increased dangers and shorter duration of the euphoria. Yet "mainlining" coke is popular among those having previous experience with the needle, and an elaborate set of procedures for injecting the drug has developed, just as it did for heroin.

SKIN DEEP

Cocaine is sometimes applied to the genitals as a desensitizer, to prolong intercourse and retard climax.

Sprinkling cocaine on the penis or clitoris does, indeed, numb the area and delay orgasm. But the price can be high. If cocaine enters the urethra, through which urine is eliminated, it will get into the bloodstream very quickly, and probably lead to a cocaine overdose. Anyone intending to apply cocaine to the genitals must be warned: THE URETHRAL OPENING MUST BE COMPLETELY AVOIDED. COCAINE MUST NEVER BE APPLIED INSIDE THE VAGINA, or used to such an extent on the penis that it spreads throughout the vagina.

There is the danger, too, that cocaine may dry up the tissues that should remain somewhat moist in order to make intercourse enjoyable.

Another use of direct application of coke, rubbing it on the gums, has been seen among people whose nasal tissues are damaged by inhalation. The effect is slowed absorption.

But an increasingly popular method of cocaine ingestion involves mixing it with some sodium bicarbonate and holding it under the tongue. The combination releases the cocaine alkaloid very quickly, and its rapid absorption into the bloodstream is said to provide a "high" similar to that provided by freebasing.

4
A BUSINESS FOR ALL SEASONS

"It's as easy as 1-2-3!"

That's the judgment of a mid-level cocaine distributor who has never been arrested, has never (to his knowledge) been investigated, and has never even been questioned by drug enforcement authorities.

"There's nothing simpler than dealing coke," he says. "You buy. You sell. You take a percentage. You get rich."

The cocaine dealer's assessment of his own chance of being arrested is supported by prosecutors and investigators all around the country. Says the special narcotics prosecutor in New York City, where drugs account for an estimated $50 billion a year in cash transactions: "Only between 5 and 10 percent of those currently dealing in drugs on a regular basis in the city ever come close to getting caught."

As for the long list of lawyers, teachers, doctors, executives, and others who *have* been identified as drug dealers, the prosecutor adds: "There's a feeling all around town today that to get caught dealing drugs you've either got to be very, very dumb or very, very unlucky."

The U.S. Drug Enforcement Administration reports that, although cocaine arrests nearly doubled from 1979 to 1982, convictions remained about the same.

THE STORY BEGINS

The multinational cocaine business—and it *is* a business, responding to the same laws of supply and demand as any other—has its roots in the fertile soil of South America, where hundreds of thousands of Bolivian, Colombian, and Peruvian farmers own or lease small plots, or *cocals,* planted in coca.

These farmers' worries are common to any farmer's. Drought, a destructive insect or fungus, and the availability of fertilizer are all discussed over meals and in the coca fields. The *ulu* caterpillar, capable of destroying a farmer's coca crop in a matter of hours, is of particular concern in some areas, while elsewhere the battle is waged against soil erosion.

Just a decade ago, only a few regions in the Andes were considered capable of supporting the hungry coca plants. But as demand for cocaine increased, mainly in the United States, areas once ignored as too cold, too wet, or too difficult to reach were cleared for cultivation. The cocaine content of leaves harvested in many of the newly-planted coca plots is lower than that from long-established plants, but in impoverished villages where an extra few dollars can close the door to starvation, added income, however small, encourages farmers to plant wherever possible.

In established growing areas, coca leaves are harvested as often as four times yearly. Growers are careful to take only as many leaves as each plant can stand to lose without dying. A few plants, their new buds ready to open at the next rainfall, may be stripped completely, left looking like crops in Minnesota fields in the last days of winter. An experienced farmer can pluck every leaf from a coca plant in just a few seconds.

The rich green leaves are stuffed into cloth sacks, often old flour sacks, tied to the farmer's waist. He is often joined by his wife, children, and other members of his close-knit extended family, each of them bending over the plants and stuffing a sack with coca leaves.

When filled, each sack will weigh only a few pounds. A full day's work for an entire farming family in the height of a harvest will yield perhaps 50 pounds of leaves.

The crop is carried, sometimes along miles of steep, twisting trails cut into the hard clay slopes, to the farmer's simple house. There, he spreads the leaves on a terrace reserved exclusively for coca leaves, and lets them dry. If the sun shines too long, the leaves will become brittle, and bring a low price; they must be turned periodically whenever the sky is cloudless, which sometimes requires several trips away from the coca field in a single day.

THE FIRST PROCESSING

Increasingly often, the farmers themselves engage in the first steps of turning the leaves into coca paste. More than 100 kilograms of leaves are needed to make a single kilo of paste, and it is much easier to transport the paste to market than to manage the movement of huge supplies of leaves every fortnight or so. Through a relatively simple and inexpensive process, the farmers make a thick, aromatic paste containing not only cocaine, but several other alkaloids as well.

Other growers take advantage of nearby processing facilities, usually crude establishments surrounded by drums of leaves in varying stages of processing. One such lab, recently destroyed by South American anti-drug agents, was capable of producing 22,000 pounds of cocaine monthly; at another, 25,300 pounds of cocaine—worth close to a billion dollars—were seized. The farmers themselves, however, cannot hope to earn more than the equivalent of a dollar or so each day.

About a dozen farmers in a single geographic area—between two streams, or on a single mountain slope—may join together to deal exclusively with one *guia,* or guide, who will regularly visit them and purchase a few kilos of coca paste, which he will then take to a laboratory in or near a major city for further processing. In many regions, though, the farmers transport their leaves or coca paste to central marketplaces, which operate openly in villages large and small.

One such market is in La Paz, Bolivia, where on Sunday morning hectic coca dealing is reminiscent of the stock market on Wall Street. Two-hundred-pound bales of compressed coca leaves trade hands throughout the day amid traffic jams of trucks and mules bringing coca in or out.

Almost everyone is chewing coca leaves or sipping coca tea to ward off the chill—and the discomfort of the high altitude—as bargains are struck, delivery schedules set, and strangers are eyed suspiciously. An ever-present danger is the possibility that undercover American antidrug agents are trying to discover details about coca shipments in order to intercept them when the drug arrives in Miami, New York, or Los Angeles.

Buyers of large supplies deliver the leaves to laboratories for processing into paste and even purer cocaine, and begin arranging with professional smugglers—the upper echelon of the cocaine business—to ship the drug to the United States and around the world. The end product of their purchases—the street coke—is dependent in part on the quantity of paste bought through middlemen directly from farmers.

THE PAYOFFS

It is usually at the marketplace level of the industry where payoffs are negotiated with government officials, police and military authorities, and others with the capacity to hinder the cocaine trade.

In Bolivia, cocaine has been so closely interlinked with the government for so long that some observers doubt whether there is any meaningful difference between the government and those controlling the drug industry. Roughly $800 million yearly is earned by Bolivia from exports of tin, its major product. Cocaine, by comparison, earns the nation an estimated $8 *billion*.

So generous has cocaine been to government and military leaders, middlemen, and even farmers, that thousands of acres of Bolivia, Colombia, and Peru are every month being converted from food crops—and even marijuana—to coca bushes. One report issued by the National Association of Financial Institutions in Colombia, for example, confirmed the change in planting patterns and, while expressing concern about the reduction in essential foodstuffs available to the population, nevertheless said the government understands the change, since coca leaves provide 400 percent more income than vegetables.

Washington has for several years tried reaching agreement with one South American government or another to halt the flow of cocaine and marijuana. The United States has offered economic incentives and low-interest loans, but most cocaine executives are suspicious of White House motives.

Why stop growing marijuana in the Andes, they wonder, except to improve the plant's economic success in California? And why put a stop to cocaine—so vital to private and governmental economies in the south—when North Americans themselves are such avid enthusiasts of the drug?

Drug traffickers look with bewilderment at Mexico's agreement allowing the United States to spray its marijuana crop with the potentially deadly herbicide paraquat, while in the U.S., the chemical is hardly ever permitted and less effective methods are used to destroy marijuana. They see this as yet another of Uncle Sam's double standards, and worry about the gringo's motives in their own countries.

American efforts to reduce cocaine production have had some success in Colombia, where the government established a high-level task force to wipe out coca plantations. After the 1984 assassination of task force head Justice Minister Rodrigo Lara Bonilla, presumably at the hands of cocaine dealers, President Belisario Betancur expanded his crackdown on cocaine. At about the same time, Colombia and Venezuela agreed to join forces against drug trafficking along their border, where guerrilla forces are hired to protect drug traffickers.

In Peru, meanwhile, coca production continues, despite millions of dollars spent by Washington on special Peruvian military units trained to track down and destroy processing facilities and coca farms.

RUNNING COKE...

The most secretive individuals along the cocaine road from South to North America are smugglers. While a tourist can comfortably chat with growers, middlemen, and government officials in La Paz about cocaine, even the most effective undercover agent has trouble passing through the narrowest part of the cocaine hourglass. Big-time smuggling, despite its pervasiveness, is wrapped in black shrouds.

But some details about how it's done emerge through court documents and interviews with antidrug agents.

By Air...

A large percentage of illicit cocaine is brought into the United States by air. Large bags of processed cocaine hydrochloride, weighing upwards of 500 pounds, are trucked to military or commercial airports and loaded onto privately owned, long-range airplanes for flights north.

Some smugglers own entire fleets of aircraft, and are careful to purchase only those planes capable of landing on small fields or out-of-the-way roads, in darkness, with no air controllers to guide their way. Cockpit equipment is often as sophisticated as that found in the best fighter jets of the U.S. Air Force.

Pilots can earn tens of thousands of dollars for a single flight, ample compensation for the chances they take. A single misstep, a sole navigational miscalculation, and they will not find the particular 500-foot-long stretch of land where they, and their tons of cocaine, are expected.

They cannot use the radio to send a Mayday message, since they are not supposed to be *in* the air. They have not filed flight plans and would certainly be arrested upon landing if air traffic officials knew their location.

But few ever encounter trouble. Their planes land, their cargos are unloaded, and they're back in the air in minutes, with extra fuel tanks to make possible the long return flight to South America.

. . . And By Sea

Some smugglers prefer using ships to move their cocaine north. Ships offer some important advantages over aircraft: they can off-load cocaine at ports farther north than planes can fly without having to worry about refueling or radar; they can carry large amounts of the drug without concern for its weight; and, unless suspicion—perhaps brought on by an informer's tip—forces a particularly detailed search, most ocean-going vessels provide thousands of hiding places where drugs could go unnoticed in routine checks.

The cocaine usually is flown (and occasionally trucked) from near its South American source to one of the numerous ports where ships regularly sail up the Pacific to California, or north across the Caribbean to the Gulf of Mexico, and from there up the Eastern seaboard.

After a few days at sea, the ships usually rendezvous with smaller craft capable of reaching shallow-water harbors or private boat docks under the smugglers' control. This is the most hazardous part of the transportation route, since U.S. Coast Guard patrols are constantly on the lookout for large ships in close proximity to small boats. The smugglers frequently attach heavy weights or chains to their illicit cargos so that, at the first sign of Coast Guard interest, they can toss the drugs overboard where they will never be found. Packages of cocaine, marijuana, and other drugs have been known to wash up on beaches as far north as New York's Long Island, the apparent result of poorly attached weights.

To avoid Coast Guard patrols, smugglers often wait in Cuban waters until their innocent-looking patrol boats uncover a safe route to Florida. Cuba allows the drug-running in return for payments as high as $500,000 in hard currency per shipment.

Under the eye of heavily armed escorts, the cocaine is off-loaded from the small boats into waiting vans or station wagons, and swiftly moved to a nearby safe house. There, it is weighed and carefully examined, perhaps for the first time, by a distributor purchasing the drug at wholesale prices.

Division and Distribution

Until the packages of cocaine are precisely inventoried on North American soil, the drug has usually not been "cut," at least not with the approval of its purchasers. But pilots, ship captains, and others involved in its transportation do not hesitate to take advantage of any opportunity to substitute a less valuable chemical for a few pounds of coke, and keep the pure cocaine as a "tip" for their work.

The ultimate street value of each cocaine shipment is determined at the safe house. Elaborate chemical tests are sometimes conducted, but wholesalers more often rely on the look, taste, and smell of the white powder to decide on its worth. If there's doubt, they may perform a foil burn test or a bleach test to confirm or refute their suspicions. Only a small degree of adulteration is permitted.

But if the "cocaine" turns out to be more sugar than coke, the distributor will try to trace its route back to South America and eliminate anyone suspected of making large cuts. This is difficult, considering the secretive nature of smuggling, and wholesale violence is frequently the distributor's only recourse.

Entire smuggling enterprises—a dozen or more

individuals—have been wiped out by distributors angered over the delivery of adulterated cocaine. Weapons found by police investigating vicious cocaine-related murders include the world's most advanced small arms, hand grenades, elaborate bombs, and anti-tank rockets and rocket launchers.

Coke violence is not limited to those directly involved in the drug. A 1982 dispute of unknown origin in Queens, N.Y., ended in the slaughter of a 29-year-old South American cocaine dealer, his wife, their four-month-old son, and an eighteen-month-old daughter. In their home, police found 140 pounds of cocaine, an arsenal of weapons, and close to a million dollars in cash.

Cocaine-related mayhem is viewed by Miami police as the leading cause of that city's high murder rate, with various groups of smugglers and distributors battling for territory, and waging a private war of honor, on the city's streets.

After testing, a wholesaler's cocaine cache is divided into packets of several kilograms each, which are transported around the country by plane, car, bus, or train. The rail lines linking Florida with New York City are so often used for cocaine shipments that any train heading north is likely to be dubbed the "Cocaine Express" by officials trying to check it for drug supplies.

Once a particular shipment of coke—perhaps 10 kilos—reaches its destination in the hands of a wholesaler, it is divided among several major distributors. At the distributor level, the drug usually is subject to its first significant cuts, of amphetamine, mannitol, sugar, caffeine, or some other substance favored by the distributors and those who will next be involved with the drug, the cocaine dealers.

While wholesalers are usually men and women with close personal and professional ties to their South American associates, and follow the coke industry much like the executives of any other business keep track of events affecting their product overseas, both distributors and dealers are somewhat removed from normal business uncertainties, such as the weather in a specific region of the Andes, or South American governments' drug negotiations. While the movement of antidrug agents in Peru or Bolivia is of vital interest to growers and wholesalers, it seldom affects traffickers farther north unless they have limited themselves to buying from a single cocaine supplier. Their interests instead are how much to cut the drug while insuring maximum profit, in what cities and states the cocaine will sell most quickly, which local police departments threaten them most seriously, and—perhaps more important—how much of the drug they themselves can take as a part of their profit.

Major dealers who handle cocaine by the kilo, and less important dealers who buy only a few ounces at a time for resale, are often cocaine users as well. They gain a supply for their own use by cutting the coke still further, or "short-weighting" their customers. A 15-ounce "pound" of cocaine is not unusual, nor is an eventual street purchase of a "gram" weighing only nine-tenths of a gram.

A dealer-user's common purchase is a quarter-ounce of cocaine, about seven grams. It will be packaged for sale in "bindles" of folded paper or light cardboard (such as a 3 x 5 index card) each holding a gram, or a half-gram, of coke. The dealer-user will retain perhaps two grams for personal use, and the retained cocaine may constitute his sole profit.

Big-time smuggling is not the only way for cocaine to enter the United States. Individuals import the drug as well, hiding a pound or so in their suitcases, clothing, or in stuffed dolls purchased abroad and brought into the country past unsuspecting customs agents.

It is a route also favored by some professional smugglers who are willing to pay couriers thousands of dollars for their risks of being caught and prosecuted. These are the couriers, or "mules," who swallow cocaine wrapped in condoms tied tight with dental floss, and who from time to time suffer from overdoses when a packet bursts in the digestive system.

Most amateur smugglers are novices who use the drug themselves, or foresee fantastic profits from a few quick trips to Peru or Bolivia. Almost anyone can purchase a kilo or so of cocaine close to its source. And the cost there is substantially lower than here, permitting huge markups after the drug is imported.

A 58-year-old woman was arrested for trying to get past customs agents at Kennedy Airport with a few ounces of cocaine hidden under her girdle. A man was taken into custody when coke was found hidden inside his wooden leg. A "nun" was charged with smuggling after cocaine was found stashed beneath her habit.

Relatively small cocaine shipments sometimes enter the country in normal international mails, in diplomatic pouches, in unattended crates addressed to legitimate businesses and marked "coffee" or "blue jeans." One supply was hidden in a large shipment of South American cut flowers, a rarely suspect commodity frequently sent north.

For every kilogram of coke smuggled by an individual amateur or small-time professional, a hundred kilos find their way to the streets of big cities, and the unpaved roads of rural America, via major importers.

The arrest of a middle-aged, middle-class man or woman who vacationed in Peru and brought back a year's supply of cocaine for personal use indicates cocaine's incredible popularity here among a wider and wider segment of the population. And the seizure of 1,600 pounds of almost pure cocaine in an East Coast restaurant parking lot—or a quarter of a ton hidden on board a ship just docked in San Francisco—demonstrates the size of the smuggling endeavor.

WHERE THE MONEY GOES

Cocaine generates cash like nothing else in the world.

If the profits of America's 500 largest corporations are added together, they barely equal the total amount of cash generated each year by illegal drugs, which the Federal Drug Enforcement Administration says amounts to more than $79 *billion* annually.

An enormous amount of that drug money—perhaps as much as half—stems from cocaine.

And there are no taxes. No reporting of income. No paperwork.

Just cash. Mountains of it.

So much cash, in fact, that some smugglers and wholesalers don't even bother counting their money. Instead, they weigh it, just as they weigh their cocaine. A certain number of five dollar bills, or tens or twenties, equals a certain amount of money. If their scales are a trifle miscalibrated, and they lose, say, $50,000 on a transaction, that's no cause for concern. They deal in the millions of dollars. A few thousand hardly matters.

What matters, though, is what they *do* with the cash. Sizeable bank deposits are closely monitored under federal law. Banks are required to report to the Treasury Department the names and social security numbers of those depositing $10,000 or more in cash. Stock and bond investments are handled in a similar fashion. Even buying a new home requires paperwork and financial reporting, so is off-limits to the person overburdened with cocaine cash.

More often than not, the money is "washed" through banks located in countries whose most important product is financial secrecy: the Cayman Islands, the Bahamas, Panama, and other island nations dotting the Caribbean. Switzerland, formerly the bank secrecy haven of first resort, has signed too many treaties with the U.S. permitting American authorities access to information about peculiar deposits to be attractive to drug capital.

Sometimes the money is deposited directly into American banks. It has been estimated that sixty to seventy banks in southern Florida have knowingly, or unwittingly, received drug deposits. It is widely believed—and for the most part proven—that some banks in every major American city have been involved with accepting drug money. They manage this by "interpreting" banking rules loosely, and granting special customers an exemption from reporting requirements.

When cocaine smugglers left Florida, after learning of increased Coast Guard patrols off the Florida shores, and headed for California, they left their illegal surplus cash in Florida banks; the accounts have remained stagnant since 1980. But in California, where banks reported a deficit of $300 million in 1980, they recorded a net gain two years later of $1 billion.

MAKING IT LEGAL?

Money-washing is relatively simple. The cash itself—in suitcases, cloth bags, large pockets—is physically transported to a temporary banking refuge and deposited. The "bank" may be nothing more than a tiny office and a postal box number, but nothing more is required; the cash is transferred to a secure vault, and its availability is cabled to a more legitimate bank elsewhere.

The depositor then relies on his hidden bank account for "loans," or above-board transfers to his own business or bank in New York, California, Florida, Texas, Louisiana, or anywhere else. The origin of the funds becomes impossible to trace since inquiries by American government authorities are met by stony silence.

Once the funds are returned to their owners, they can be declared on income tax forms as legal "loans," "gifts," or "investments" from unnamed foreign sources. And the money can then be safely spent.

Federal officials say they have been uncovering laundering operations, on a regular basis, that process close to $1 million daily, creating "worldwide ramifications," according to one official.

One 37-year-old New Yorker deeply involved in the cocaine trade bought an entire disco for $1.5 million—in cash—simply because he didn't like the service and wanted to fire the workers. When he was murdered, presumably in a row over cocaine, officials learned he had also purchased a few other "toys" with his coke dollars, including a helicopter, two other aircraft, Rolls-Royce and Mercedes automobiles, and a yacht.

Art masterpieces . . . elegant homes . . . fancy cars, boats and planes . . . all are available for cocaine money. Along with legitimate businesses both large and small.

The arrest of automaker John De Lorean, on charges that he tried setting up a $24-million international cocaine smuggling ring to bail out his financially faltering car company, sent earthquake-sized tremors through the Western world's financial community. If such a huge business, and such a prominent corporate leader, could allegedly be involved in cocaine, then what industry was immune?

Although the De Lorean case was still working its way through the courts as this book went to press, it served to point out that *no* industry can be completely sure of immunity from involvement with cocaine money. Even the most legitimate-appearing business arrangement might be supported by illicit drug profits.

Financial advisors at the respected Wall Street investment firm of Donaldson, Lufkin & Jenrette were amazed not long ago when a single brokerage account suddenly showed unusual activity. Fully $38 million was moved through the account in a brief two months. The firm notified government officials of the odd manipulations, and several Colombians were quickly arrested. Had the investors handled their money with more savvy, they would most likely be free today.

The "cocaine cupcake caper" is another example of the close ties between coke and corporations. A major bakery was found to be selling cupcakes for $40,000 each, cash on delivery. The company, investigators learned, was in reality a major cocaine distribution center, apparently financed with drug money.

From coast to coast, businesses of every kind are being built on cocaine dollars. A suburban industrial complex near Chicago . . . a Midwestern resort . . . an office building in New York . . . all could put a few grams of cocaine in their cornerstones, to symbolize their origins.

"Any company can be bought with drug money," said a federal investigator, "because there's absolutely no way to be sure it *is* drug money."

5
THE COKE TEST

The way cocaine acts in bleach has become a well-known method of testing the purity of cocaine.

Although commonly called the "Clorox" test, any laundry bleach can be used if it contains 5.25 percent (by weight) sodium hypochlorite, a common bleaching chemical. The brand name of just one widely available bleaching agent was applied to the cocaine test late in the '60s, and the "Clorox" test has come to mean a cocaine test performed with any similar household bleach.

WHY A BLEACH TEST?

Laundry bleach is inexpensive and easily available.

This fact, along with a unique interaction with cocaine and common coke "cuts," has made the use of bleach a popular method for quickly determining the purity of a purchase. All the material needed for this test is easily carried in a pocket, purse, or small parcel; elaborate equipment is not needed.

HOW THE TEST IS CONDUCTED

The behavior of cocaine when it has been cut—the residue it leaves behind and the kind of path it makes through the bleach—provides an indication of its purity and, if impure, the most likely cutting agents.

A tiny quantity of highly refined cocaine, when dropped into a glass of bleach, hesitates on the surface for a few seconds, then slowly falls to the bottom of the glass in milky whisps like trails of white smoke.

Near-pure cocaine leaves no residue on the bottom of the glass, and only a small, barely noticeable oily film on the surface of the bleach.

In conducting the test, a clear glass about six inches high is used. It has to be spotlessly clean and completely dry before the bleach is poured into it. The bleach is used at room temperature, about 70 degrees Fahrenheit, and has to be allowed to stand until the liquid is totally still.

A small, finely chopped sample of cocaine—about 10 milligrams—is dropped from a clean razor blade or sharp knife on top of the bleach in the middle of the glass.

The path the sample takes as it falls through the bleach is the determining factor. How long does it take to fall? Is the path straight, or curly? Milky white, or tinted with color? What shape and color is the residue left on top of the bleach? On the bottom of the glass? Did the sample dissolve completely, or are there tiny particles still intact?

Cocaine will begin to fall through the bleach after resting on the surface for perhaps three or four seconds. Within about ten seconds, it will be almost completely dissolved, and can be seen drifting through the liquid in an almost graceful manner. Any part of the sample acting differently is not cocaine, but one of several "cuts" used to dilute the drug.

WHAT "CUTS" CAN BE SEEN?

The "Clorox" test is most effective in detecting adulterants and dilutants added to the cocaine in powdered form.

COCAINE CUTS

These substances are commonly used to adulterate, or lessen, the amount of cocaine present in a sample—thereby "stretching" the amount to be sold or consumed.

Sugars

Mannitol (a baby laxative)
Lactose (milk sugar)
Glucose
Dextrose
Inositol
Sucrose

Salts

Lidocaine (psychoactive drug)
Procaine (" ")
Tetracaine (" ")

Others

Acetaminophen
Amphetamine
Ascorbic Acid
Aspirin
Benzocaine
Boric Acid
Butacaine
Caffeine
Calcium
Cornstarch
Ephedrine
Flour
Heroin
Ketamine
Magnesium sulfate
Phenylpropanolamine
Talc

The adulterants with some psychoactive properties which the test can pinpoint include lidocaine, caffeine, ephedrine, benzocaine, and phenylpropanolamine.

Dilutants, the inactive ingredients which may show up in the test, can include mannitol, lactose, dextrose, sucrose, talc, flour, and cornstarch.

Other substances whose presence the bleach test can indicate are amphetamine, procaine, tetracaine, butacaine, acetaminophen, ascorbic acid, boric acid, calcium, heroin, magnesium sulfate, quinine, sodium bicarbonate, methaqualone, and pemoline. Traces of any of these ingredients may find their way into a cocaine sample either deliberately or by accident.

A compound known as "rock crystal," the so-called legal alternative to cocaine, may also be disclosed; it is made of mannitol, benzocaine, and procaine, and is often used to dilute cocaine prior to sale on the street. Rock crystal is also sometimes sold as a cocaine substitute, rather than a "cut."

All these chemicals and compounds leave distinct residues in a glass of bleach. Some fail completely to fall through the liquid, producing instead a patch of clear or colored oil on top of the bleach, sometimes sprinkled with suspended powder. Others drop like dozens of minuscule pebbles straight to the bottom of the glass, where they quickly turn brown or dark green.

Samples with some cocaine content will show both characteristics: the cocaine will dissolve completely, while the "cut" will act differently, either floating on the bleach or dropping quickly to the bottom. By comparing the proportions of dissolved material with the rest of the sample, it is possible to estimate how much of the overall sample is actually cocaine.

ELUDING THE "CLOROX" TEST

When the bleach test first became known in the cocaine underground, it provided users with quick, accurate answers to their questions about purity. But in the illicit cocaine marketplace, suppliers try to keep current with consumer awareness and, where possible, find ways to defeat it.

Almost as fast as the test's popularity grew, cocaine distributors, and others higher up in the production and smuggling chain, sought ways to counteract the test. New methods to cut cocaine are constantly being developed to evade the "Clorox" test. To reduce the effectiveness of the test, some coke suppliers even began introducing other ingredients earlier in the refining process, which makes them increasingly difficult to detect with bleach.

IS THE TEST STILL VALID?

Yes! Even though the bleach test cannot be an absolute measure of cocaine's purity, it remains the simplest, cheapest, fastest, and safest way for a cocaine buyer to determine with any degree of certainty the purity of each purchase.

An enormous amount of cocaine is still cut in the traditional manner, with ingredients such as sugars, local anesthetics, and amphetamine, all of which are visible in bleach.

The interpretation of the results of the "Clorox" test is, of course, subjective. There is no absolute chart of colors, or scale of residue, against which to compare the results of each cocaine sample tested. Different testers may well reach different conclusions as to the purity of a particular pinch of coke. A practiced eye and what it observes are key factors in deciding whether someone will take the chance and buy, or use, a specific supply of cocaine.

As with any chemical analysis, results of several separate tests, considered together, are more conclusive than the result of a single test. A number of variables can invalidate one test: a smudged glass, unexpected vibrations, too warm (or cold) bleach, etc. Whenever possible, samples from the same supply of cocaine are studied in bleach at least twice, and more reliably three times.

The bleach test is sometimes combined with another cocaine test, the "foil burn," to show a sample's purity more clearly. In this test a small sample of cocaine is put on a piece of household aluminum foil and held over a flame until the sample melts. This may provide added evidence of the purity and indicate the kind of "cut" used, since pure cocaine will melt evenly into a uniform puddle with little color. Any "cut" will melt either faster, or slower, than the cocaine, and result in brown, gray, or greenish residue.

THE COLOR PLATES

The Coke Book's photo section contains color plates showing cocaine and various cocaine cuts undergoing the bleach test.

Some of the photographs depict the possession and testing of cocaine under approved laboratory conditions. Possession and testing without prescription or approval would be illegal.

Plates A, B, C and **D** illustrate the action of a small amount of pure cocaine when dropped into a glass of household bleach. Within seconds, wisps of cocaine fall partway through the bleach; a few seconds later some of it reaches the bottom of the glass. By 31 seconds, most of the sample is suspended in the liquid, and shortly afterwards begins to disappear.

Plates E and **F** demonstrate the typical action of "Synth Coke," sold at so-called "head shops" around the country as well as on the street. Although the sample used for these photos could "beat the Clorox test," according to the package, the way it acts in bleach demonstrates otherwise. The product contains no cocaine, and although it is promoted as "incense," uninformed buyers apparently believe they are purchasing a powerful stimulant.

Plates G and **H** show a genuine non-cocaine stimulant, D-Amphetamine, commonly called "speed." While dangerous if abused, it is not as potent as coke. Because D-Amphetamine is so much less expensive than cocaine, yet still provides users with a substantial level of stimulation, it is a popular cocaine cut.

Plates I, **J**, **K**, and **L** show how two other common cuts, lactose (milk sugar) and mannitol (a baby laxative), act in bleach. Both are sold at health food stores, pharmacies, and "head shops."

Plates M, **N**, **O**, and **P**: "Rock Crystal" and "Pseudocaine" are, like "Synth Coke," generally marketed as "incense—*not fit for human consumption*." The cocaine-free "Rock Crystal" should not be confused with "rock" or "Bolivian rock," a crudely refined and extremely potent substance containing a large amount of cocaine.

"Synth Coke," "Rock Crystal," and "Pseudocaine" (all brand names) usually contain varying amounts of ingredients such as caffeine, procaine, and/or benzocaine, which may give users a few minutes of mild stimulation, or numb the nose or tongue after use. When ground into fine powder, they are visually difficult to distinguish from genuine cocaine crystals. These and other cuts often comprise the bulk of a "cocaine" purchase.

The pictures in the photo insert were photographed under the auspices of Mark S. Gold, M.D., Director of Research, Fair Oaks Hospital, Summit, New Jersey. All photographs were taken at The Psychiatric Diagnostic Laboratories of America, Inc. facility in Summit, New Jersey.

6
THE COCAINE PROFILE

Throughout its history, cocaine has been a drug of both promise and disappointment.

Regardless of whether its medical or recreational use is examined, an important chemical which first appeared to be a powerfully positive substance is now fully recognized as having destructive capabilities far more significant than its outdated medical usefulness.

COKE ROOTS

The plants which produce cocaine have always been an important cash crop. Coca bushes, in fact, may well be the most valuable, naturally occurring plants in the world. Other plants generating substantial international trade—corn and wheat, for example—are far from their genetic origins, after centuries of manipulation to develop improved strains. Coca plants cultivated today are almost identical to their ancestors millions of years ago.

As much as 77 million pounds—38,000 *tons*—of dried coca leaves are produced each year in Bolivia alone, three times more than the country produced a mere decade ago. And Bolivia is not the world's sole source of cocaine.

Peru's coca-leaf production stands today at 66 million pounds annually, and other South American countries, seeing their neighbors' enormous profits from the plant, have also enthusiastically jumped aboard the cocaine railroad.

The money generated by cocaine is so great, say experts, that entire nations owe their economic existence to the drug, governments rise and fall based on their cocaine fortunes, and the international banking world could suffer a severe blow if an incurable blight suddenly struck every coca plant on earth.

Just what is this phenomenally valuable plant?

The coca plant—*Erythroxylum coca*—is indigenous to the eastern Andes mountains of South America, where today it is most commonly cultivated at elevations between 500 and 1,500 meters.

The plant is thought to have emerged long before the first human—or humanlike creature—walked the earth. The fourteen alkaloids in its leaves—cocaine is but one of these—probably evolved as chemical defenses to ward off animals anticipating a good meal of fresh greenery. Coca remains today relatively free of insect pests, and grazing animals seldom bother the plants.

Some 250 distinct species of coca have been identified, almost all growing in the same South American *montaña*. But only a few are laden with the cocaine alkaloid. One alkaloid appears to be as successful as another in giving a memorable bad taste to herbivores.

Even in its native mineral-rich clay soil, coca almost never is allowed to grow unattended; the leaves are too valuable a commodity to be far from the hand of man.

With careful tending, coca has been grown in Southeast Asia, central Europe, and the United States, but never in such quantities to make any of these regions a major source of cocaine. In the early 1900s, Dutch farmers on the Indonesian island of Java grew coca commercially using up-to-date agricultural techniques, but their business failed when the price of coca leaves dropped precipitously in the 1920s, as cocaine's dangers became apparent.

Contrary to common myths, the plant is related to neither the stubby tree providing chocolate (*Theobroma cacao*) nor the coconut palm (*Cocos nucifera*), despite the similar sounds of their scientific names.

Coca is a medium-sized shrub which will reach three or four meters in height if left to grow wild. The leaves of most species are distinguished by two parallel lines on their underside. Some varieties smell like hay, while others have the aroma of wintergreen. Propagation is by seed alone with most species, but a few reproduce equally well by cuttings.

Of the 250 varieties of coca, only two possess enough cocaine to have any economic value to farmers. These two varieties are planted in hillside rows where rainfall is abundant and temperatures are moderate. They are kept well trimmed to make harvesting as easy as possible.

First seriously cultivated in Bolivia, the coca plant there is popularly called *huanuco*. Its leaves contain between 0.5 and 1.0 percent alkaloids, dominated by cocaine.

Colombia was another early site of commercial coca cultivation, and a variety grown there, *E. novogranatense*, referred to the country's Spanish name, *Nueva Grenada*. Its leaves contain between 1.0 and 2.5 percent alkaloids, and seldom more than half of that is cocaine. The species prefers less water and more sunshine, and adapts well to a variety of climates. Coca production is now illegal in Colombia (although native Indians continue growing and using the plant), but the country has become a major distribution center.

Cocaine extracted from Peruvian plants, similar to *E. novogranatense*, is known as "Trujillo Coke," after the coastal region where it is grown. The leaves are slightly thicker than other varieties, but smaller and narrower.

According to botanist Timothy Plowman of Chicago's Field Museum of Natural History, the Peruvian coca is "much desired by the pharmaceutical industry because of its superior flavor and shipping properties." Hundreds of tons of Peruvian coca leaves a year, he says, "are still exported from Trujillo to New York for preparation of extracts used in the manufacture of Coca-Cola," which is cocaine-free, the cocaine itself having been already extracted for sale legally to the pharmaceutical industry.

While most varieties of the coca plant grow well in their native climates with relatively little intervention, the Peruvian strain is "never found growing outside of cultivation," says Plowman, "since it depends upon at least some irrigation for continued survival. . . ."

Until colonial times, coca proliferated in Ecuador, where the oldest evidence of its use has been found. Researchers believe its disappearance there was brought about by early government and religious edicts discouraging the plant's use.

EARLY USES

South America's earliest inhabitants believed coca cleared their minds, elevated their moods, gave them energy, helped digestion, suppressed their appetites, promoted longevity, and cured "altitude sickness." They regarded the plant as "a gift from heaven to better the lives of people on earth," says noted drug expert Andrew Weil, M.D.

Chewing coca leaves could have begun as early as 5000 B.C., when most South American wildlife had been hunted to the brink of extinction, and early inhabitants struggled to find new food sources. Indeed, the nutritional benefits of coca leaves might have made them a significant part of the everyday diet. One hundred grams of coca leaves contain 305 calories, nearly 19 grams of protein, more than 40 grams of carbohydrates, and enough calcium, iron, phosphorus, and vitamins A, B_2, and E to satisfy the U.S. government's recommended dietary allowances.

The leaves were probably eaten then much as they are today: chewed to softness, mixed in the mouth with a pinch of lime from the ashes of burned plants (which releases the cocaine), then held between cheek and tongue and sucked.

Archaeological evidence indicates that a liquid coca-leaf compound may have first been used as a local anesthetic as long ago as 1500 B.C., when surgical holes were bored into the heads of Indians.

During the time of the Incas, the coca plant was accorded a "sacred" status. It was used in religious rituals by priests, and even placed into the mouths of the dead to "ease the journey into the next world." The leaves were a good-luck charm to attract love and wealth, and were part of initiation rites and weddings.

Together with other plants considered vital to Inca life—such as maize and quinine—coca was thought to have a divine essence known as the plant's "mother." Renowned in stories and myths, "Mama Coca" was depicted as a beautiful woman. An Inca ruler even named his queen Mama Coca.

Where coca was sacred, it was not widely available to the common Indian, except in ceremonies and as medicine. Its daily use remained restricted until the Spanish conquest, which upset traditional religious taboos as well as the food economy. After 1536, use of the leaves spread quickly throughout a malnourished population, probably because it suppressed the appetites. Soon the Spaniards discovered that cultivating the plant could earn them a huge profit, and the money-making motive helped coca gain widespread distribution.

THE DRUG OF THE 1880s

Although Europeans had heard vague and mysterious tales about coca since its discovery in the New World, firsthand knowledge and serious interest in the plant were delayed for almost two hundred years.

Not until the late 18th century did detailed reports of the plant's virtues begin to spread in Europe, partly through stories brought back by sailors who had experienced the leaves while visiting South America's Pacific coast. By 1750, specimens had reached European researchers, who classified the plant according to scientific standards.

German scientist Friedrich Gaedcke is believed to have been the first, in 1855, to isolate the chief alkaloid in coca. He originally named it erythroxyline. In 1860 Albert Niemann isolated and named the coca alkaloid "cocaine" and noted its numbing effect on the tongue. Almost immediately, cocaine became popular among Europeans both as a medicine and a pleasure drug.

Just a few years later, Corsican chemist Angelo Mariani introduced the public to the first coca-containing elixir, "Vin Mariani." With an entrepreneurial spirit unheard of a century ago—tireless promotion, the collection of an incredible array of testimonials, and the support of a fanatic following—the chemist came even closer than Timothy Leary to "turning on" the world.

The popularity of Vin Mariani, with its cure-all reputation, attracted statements of support from the likes of Thomas Edison and Pope Leo XIII. "Solar rays in bottles," proclaimed the founder of the French Society of Astronomers. "So often restored my strength," announced composer Charles Gounod. Even U.S. President William McKinley sent a note of thanks to Mariani for a case of the famous tonic.

PRAISE FOR VIN MARIANI

THOMAS ALVA EDISON: "Monsieur Mariani, I take pleasure in sending you one of my photographs for publication in your Album. Yours very truly."

CAMILLE FLAMMARION (an astronomer who founded the French Society of Astronomers): "Solar rays in bottles."

CHARLES GOUNOD (composer of symphonies and operas): "To my good friend Mariani, beneficial revealer of this admirable coca wine from Peru, which has so often restored my strength."

CARDINAL LAVIGERIE: "Your coca from America gave my European priests the strength to civilise Asia and Africa."

POPE LEO XIII, in a message conveyed through a cardinal: "Rome, January 2, 1898. His Holiness has deigned to commission me to thank the distinguished donor in His holy name, and to demonstrate His gratitude in a material way as well. His Holiness does me the honour of presenting Mr. Mariani with a gold medal containing His venerable coat-of-arms."

WILLIAM McKINLEY (President of the United States): "Executive Mansion, Washington, June 14, 1898. My dear Sir, Please accept thanks on the President's behalf and on my own for your courtesy in sending a case of the celebrated Vin Mariani, with whose tonic virtues I am already acquainted, and will be happy to avail myself of in the future as occasion may require. Very truly yours, John Addison Porter, Secretary to the President."

AUGUSTE RODIN: "To Mariani, who spreads coca. Your friend."

JULES VERNE: "Since a single bottle of Mariani's extraordinary coca wine guarantees a lifetime of a hundred years, I shall be obliged to live until the year 2700! Well, I have no objections! Yours very gratefully."

Source: Lee, David. *Cocaine Handbook: An Essential Reference.* Berkeley, California: And/Or Press, Inc. 1981.

In 1886, a "health drink" much like Vin Mariani—but without the wine—came on the scene. Called Coca-Cola, it was the predecessor of today's popular soft drink and "the first generally advertised product that directed people to a drug store," according to researcher-author Robert Wilson. The beverage was served at soda fountains across the country, and its nickname, coke, became the popular name of the drink's active ingredient.

Within a few years there were dozens of similar beverages available to the general public, all containing cocaine. Men, women, and children alike visited drug stores for a "pick-me-up" of soda laced with cocaine.

Other popular preparations containing cocaine included a variety of ointments, and the popular slow-burning "Coca Leaf Smoke Ball," an "approved cure" for asthma, whooping cough, snoring, "throat deafness," and other poorly defined ailments. "Recommended by leading physicians," went the advertising copy, adding: "A ball will last a family several months."

Cocaine atomizer inhalants also became popular for weaning tobacco smokers of nicotine and for treating youngsters with whooping cough.

THE FREUD CONNECTION

Throughout the 1880s, medical enthusiasm for cocaine rose steadily. Sigmund Freud's landmark 1884 paper, *On Coca,* described the drug's effects on himself, and outlined several major uses for cocaine: as a stimulant, for digestive disorders, to treat morphine and alcohol addiction, and asthma, as an aphrodisiac, and as a local anesthetic. Only the last of these proved to be enduring in medical circles.

Although Freud mentioned in passing that excessive cocaine use could cause "physical and intellectual decadence," weakness, emaciation, and "moral depravity," the founder of modern psychotherapy was more interested in coke's medicinal potential. Used in moderation, he concluded, cocaine was "more likely to promote health than impair it."

Firmly convinced of cocaine's benefits, Freud treated the morphine habit of his physician friend Ernst von Fleischl-Marxow by substituting cocaine for the supposedly more dangerous morphine. But von Fleischl's cocaine use got out of hand, and he began to suffer from toxic symptoms. "The most frightful night" of von Fleischl's life, Freud later wrote, was caused by a cocaine overdose.

While expressing sorrow and guilt over his role in a close friend's suffering, Freud nevertheless continued experimenting with, and writing about, cocaine, but concentrated on its psychoactive properties, rather than its anesthetic uses. Largely influenced by Freud's work, in 1885 the Parke Davis company—with some qualifications—declared cocaine "the most important therapeutic discovery of the age."

Credit for using cocaine as an anesthetic deservedly goes to Carl Koller, an associate of Freud's at Vienna General Hospital, who supported the drug for ophthalmic procedures. Until then, eye operations like cataract removals had been performed without any anesthesia whatsoever; they were extremely painful and difficult to accomplish. Koller's successful use of cocaine to anesthetize a patient's eye was quickly extended to nose, throat, gynecological, urinary, and dental procedures.

Almost simultaneously, American physician William Stewart Halsted of Johns Hopkins—the "father of modern surgery"—developed a technique of using the drug as a "neural block," which permitted specific regions of the body to be anesthetized. Soon thereafter, cocaine was injected as a spinal block as well, and it was the only local anesthesia available until the discovery of novocaine in 1899.

Cocaine was prescribed as a system-wide stimulant, as a bromide for seasickness, head colds, and "hysterical depression," and as a preventative for female masturbation.

In his 1901 book *Peru: A History of Coca,* W. Gorden Mortimer advised cocaine as a cure for "neurasthenia," a then-recognized combination of ailments including headache, digestive problems, the inability to work, loss of sexual desire, muscle weakness and stiffness, back pain, insomnia, and "hypocondrial views of life."

The drug found favor among singers, athletes, and physicians. Narcotics addicts were turning to cocaine by the thousands, either seeking relief from their withdrawal symptoms, or looking for a new, legal drug to enjoy.

THE BUBBLE BURSTS

At the same time that cocaine was becoming more popular, the drug's potentially toxic impact was beginning to surface.

Halsted and several of his assistants became addicted while conducting cocaine experiments; the surgeon himself was twice hospitalized—for periods totaling more than a year—because of his cocaine compulsion, and he was forced to take an extended coke-free cruise to try to cure himself. He failed, and died addicted to both cocaine and the morphine he believed would ease his cocaine problem.

Medical papers were published with warnings of cocaine intoxication and abuse among voluntary users, and telling of acute and chronic physical and psychological disturbances, including drug dependence.

Freud's support of cocaine as a cure for morphine addiction drew increased fire from medical writers. In 1887 the psychoanalyst himself, in a paper titled *Craving for and Fear of Cocaine*, called the drug "a far more dangerous enemy to health than morphine." Once substitutes became available for surgical anesthesia, cocaine's medical role was restricted to topical use, a further blow to its popularity in the community of physicians.

The American Pharmacological Association, in 1901, set up a "Committee on the Acquirement of the Drug Habit," which condemned cocaine and its manufacturers with equal vehemence.

The anti-cocaine flames were fanned even hotter by virulent racist comments by medical "experts" and inflammatory newspaper articles alike. The APA's "Drug Habit" committee ignored the fact that most well-documented cases of cocaine addiction were among white males, especially physicians, and railed instead against the supposed connection between blacks, cocaine, and crime.

"The negroes, the lower and criminal classes, are naturally the most readily influenced" by cocaine, the committee reported. A Presidential panel reached a similar conclusion, calling cocaine a devastating drug among southern blacks. The Journal of the American Medical Association wrote of blacks facing "a new form of vice," and going on "coke drunks."

One newspaper called cocaine a "potent incentive in driving the humbler negroes all over the country to abnormal crimes." Another warned that cocaine could keep criminals from dying of normally mortal wounds by providing "temporary immunity to shock." Newspapers reported frequently on murder and mayhem among the inner-city poor—most frequently blacks—"caused" by cocaine addiction. Often the violence was attributed to coke even when it was unknown what drug was responsible, or when it was clear *no* drug was involved.

By the time talk of a European war was first heard on this side of the Atlantic, most states had made cocaine a prescription medicine, requiring extensive records of its distribution and sale.

The Pure Food and Drug Act of 1906 severely restricted the use of cocaine in patent medicines and tonics. It had already been eliminated from Coca-Cola and many similar elixirs, and replaced by various flavoring agents and less controversial drugs like caffeine. But as late as 1909, nearly seventy Coca-Cola imitations—with cocaine—remained on the market. (Coca-Cola now uses South American coca leaves treated, before shipment, to remove all traces of cocaine.)

A popular movement to completely ban the use of coke swept across the country. In 1914, as events in Yugoslavia and Germany dominated the headlines, Congress passed the Harrison Narcotics Act, which put cocaine in the same category as the opiates. Its use for all but medicinal purposes was, at long last, outlawed.

COKE RENAISSANCE

"Laws are made to be broken."

In this case, the common saying couldn't be closer to the truth. The labyrinth of federal and state laws restricting cocaine forced the drug far underground, but did not eliminate its illegal use. Other drugs for anesthesia were becoming more and more popular; the introduction of amphetamine in 1932 offered an alternative stimulant; cocaine was becoming harder to find; the drug's price soared.

But although cocaine was buried, it was still alive. While public interest in cocaine waned from the '20s through the early '60s, the drug remained popular among society's mavericks, mainly well-connected entertainers and the less-respectable wealthy. It came to symbolize high-society decadence. Among the poor, its price made cocaine almost unobtainable, although some users managed to find affordable sources.

The 1960s introduced a new attitude toward illicit drugs among the large middle-class population just coming of age. Drug abuse was only one facet of the widespread changes our society experienced in the '60s, but it was one that would alter the focus and tenor of the way coke was used.

Cocaine was no longer a medical drug, since claims of health-related benefits had ceased long before. While only a few decades earlier cocaine's accepted medical uses brought about grave concern over its social impact, now its "acceptable" social use prompted the medical community to take a new, hard look at the drug's possible clinical applications.

Cocaine's psychoactive attributes were finally studied in depth, and the drug was tested as a treatment for catatonic stupor and depression, for use in mental disorders, and as a method to study paranoid schizophrenia. It was also tried, in combination with methadone and alcohol, for the treatment of terminal cancer pain.

Midway through the '70s, cocaine appeared among the middle-class as well as the rich. Its status as an illicit drug, as well as its upper-class "pedigree," gave cocaine a romantic, exclusive, and desirable aura. From schoolteachers to stockbrokers, coke was suddenly in vogue with a vengeance. Drug researchers began paying attention to its deleterious effects on a pleasure-seeking public.

Today, in the mid-'80s, the medical world is experimenting with cocaine as a treatment for everything from arthritis to cluster headaches. And the nonmedical world seems to be experimenting just as widely.

Will we ever come to fully understand all the divergent sides of this drug which more than once has run the gamut of medical and social opinion?

Whenever cocaine has come under close scrutiny, something new has been revealed about its nature, and the effects it can produce on the human body and the mind.

Only now are we beginning to acknowledge that despite all the medical studies of cocaine conducted over the past century . . . despite decades of grappling with cocaine's serious social implications . . . despite both praise and warnings about cocaine, there is still much more to learn about a drug that is at one and the same time described as a great discovery and a scourge.

A BRIEF HISTORY OF COCAINE

1500 B.C. Topical anesthesia made by combining saliva with juice from coca leaves. Medicinal and ceremonial use by Incas.

300 B.C. Puffed cheeks indicating wads of coca in mouth depicted on Peruvian and Ecuadorian grave statues. Speculation that Indians chewed coca leaves as stimulant, social ritual, and dietary supplement; and upper classes brewed tea from coca leaves.

1493–1527 Coca use among Incas mostly restricted to nobility.

1507 Letters of explorer Amerigo Vespucci mention Indian practice of chewing coca leaves.

1532–33 Spanish conquest of Peru and other areas of South America.

1551–67 Catholic bishops formally denounce coca as idolatry.

1613 Manuscript depicts unauthorized social use of coca by Indians when they were expected to work.

1750 First coca plants examined in Europe.

1786 Lamarck classifies *Erythroxylon coca,* now referred to as *Erythroxylum coca.*

1863 *Vin Mariani,* coca-containing elixir, introduced in Europe for popular consumption.

1883–85 Sigmund Freud praises cocaine. Cocaine used as anesthetic for ophthalmic surgery; as "nerve block" in major surgery; as spinal anesthetic; Robert Louis Stevenson writes *Dr. Jekyll and Mr. Hyde,* probably during cocaine treatment for tuberculosis.

1886 "Coca-Cola" introduced as "tonic for elderly people who were easily tired."

1887 Oregon passes first restrictive cocaine law.

1891 Medical journals report cocaine "poisoning."

1897–99 Cocaine used as anesthetic for amputations and surgical hernia repair. Medical journal estimates that 30 percent of American "cocainists" are doctors and dentists.

1903 Coca-Cola eliminates cocaine from soft drink.

1914 Cocaine classified with narcotics in Harrison Act, outlawing its use for all but medical purposes.

1961 U.N. Single Convention on Narcotic Drugs seeks to regulate drugs—including cocaine—worldwide.

1962 Peru warns that eradication of coca production would idle 200,000 workers.

1970 Cocaine used to treat depression and catatonic stupor, to diagnose mental disorders, to study paranoid schizophrenia, and with methadone and alcohol, to treat terminal cancer pain.

1980s Cocaine free-basing becomes popular; reports of toxic reactions increase sharply; cocaine used to treat migraine and severe headaches; employed as topical anesthetic in intranasal surgery; and available in powder and gel forms for use by physicians as topical anesthetic in ear, nose, and throat procedures.

NOTE: Adapted with permission from "A Medical Chronology of Cocaine" by Dr. George R. Gay in "You've Come a Long Way Baby! Coke Time for the New American Lady of the Eighties." *The Journal of Psychoactive Drugs,* vol. 13, no. 4 (October-December 1981).

7
THE METABOLIC TRAIL

Cocaine is today classified by the federal government—under the U.S. Comprehensive Drug Abuse and Control Act of 1970—as one of several "Schedule II" substances, drugs officially considered to have "high abuse potential with small recognized medical use." Other drugs in the same group include opium, morphine, amphetamine, and some barbiturates.

COCAINE'S PHARMACOLOGIC ACTIONS

Coke's tendency for abuse stems from the physical effects it has on a user's body, which are relatively well known, and from the less clearly understood psychological effects. The two chapters following this one—"Effects on the Body" and "Coke and the Mind"—explain in detail these aspects of cocaine. Though the reactions of body and mind to cocaine are so intertwined as to be virtually inseparable, they have been individually addressed to lead to a better grasp of the full range of cocaine's impact on anyone using the drug.

In this chapter, some clarifying pharmacologic information on coke, culled from the latest medical research, is provided.

The "pharmacology" of cocaine—of any drug, in fact—refers to its actions on a living entity—a human being, a research animal, or a single cell. What the drug does, and how the drug does it, are the basic facts needed to understand how the drug can best be used, and what risks it carries for those using it.

Research scientists look for sources of the physical

and mental reactions and unique behavior patterns which occur when a substance like cocaine is taken. What does coke do to the blood system? To the nerves? The lungs? Glands that produce chemicals essential to life? How does it affect brain waves, and why?

Researchers agree that cocaine exerts two main effects on the body—anesthetic and stimulant—and several related effects falling into each of those broad categories.

ANESTHETIC EFFECTS

Cocaine is the world's only well-studied naturally occurring anesthetic. The drug deadens sensation wherever it is applied, inside or outside the body. It acts most obviously when it touches the sensitive mucous membranes inside the nose and mouth, but it would eliminate sensation equally well inside the digestive system, or on a flesh wound.

Coke works as an anesthetic by blocking the conduction of electrical impulses within the nerve cells involved in sensory transmissions, primarily of pain. The body's motor impulses, such as those telling the muscles what to do, are not affected at the cocaine doses prescribed by physicians or usually taken for recreation. In this way, cocaine creates a localized blocking of pain, without interfering with body movement. Researchers call this kind of selective action a "differential block."

Another one of cocaine's anesthetic properties is its excellent efficiency as a vasoconstrictor; that is, the drug can slow down the flow of blood throughout the circulatory system. It is this ability that makes cocaine attractive as a topical anesthetic for some ear, nose, and throat procedures, during which physicians work on tissues rich in blood vessels; the drug slows the blood flow, while simultaneously reducing pain.

Cocaine is still sometimes used during plastic surgery, when the cocaine euphoria experienced by patients is believed to make the surgery more tolerable. Cocaine's effect in such procedures lasts between twenty and forty minutes.

STIMULANT EFFECTS

Cocaine is a powerful stimulant of the central nervous system. Whether it is swallowed, snorted, smoked, or injected, coke reaches the nervous system through the bloodstream. But if cocaine is smoked, it reaches the nervous system's most important part, the brain, by way of the lungs, which makes the drug's distribution much faster, and produces stronger reactions. The effects of coke on the nervous system are, to some extent, mediated by the user's emotional and psychological states, the temperature and humidity, and even the user's perception of his surroundings.

Cocaine's impact on the nervous system can be tracked through the brain's electrical activity. A high increase in the output of electrical energy is seen after chronic cocaine use. The chronic user's electroencephalogram (EEG), or brain-wave tracings, shows high nervous activity, which can drain the nervous system of resources it stores for other purposes. This suggests that a great input of "fuel," in the form of nutrients carried by the blood, is required by the nervous system to replenish what is expended by cocaine.

In addition to the *level* of electrical energy output, the *type* of energy is also significant. So-called "spindle activity," which is detectable on an EEG, greatly increases after cocaine use, and may be the cause of cocaine's effects as a sexual stimulant and violence increaser. The spindles signal stimulation to the area of the brain responsible for the "flight-or-fight" reaction to danger.

The overall "behavior arousal" experienced by cocaine users is believed to be partly related to the desynchronization of brain waves in one area of the brain, and the rhythmic slow activity that appears in another area of the brain.

CHEMICAL ACTIONS

Despite many years of study, researchers remain unsure about the precise way cocaine operates on a cellular level. Dr. Mark Gold, however, suggests one theoretical model that accounts for many of the drug's effects.

Norepinephrine (NE), dopamine (DA), and epinephrine (E), three of the body's natural neurotransmitters responsible for sending messages from one nerve cell to another, also act as stimulants, their stimulating actions constantly regulated by other neurotransmitters such as serotonin and ACH (Acetylcholine). Regular use of cocaine, Dr. Gold suspects, increases the rate of production and release of NE, DA, and E, while preventing the production and actions of the regulating chemicals. In this way, the body and brain react to the excess stimulation from some neurotransmitters which are not being adequately controlled by others. "The effect is like driving a car faster and faster, without having any brakes to stop it," says Dr. Gold.

First-time cocaine users sometimes report an absence of stimulation from the drug, with its effects only felt after repeated usage. This could be due, according to Dr. Gold's theoretical model, to the initial response of serotonin to cocaine. While this "controlling" neurotransmitter is eventually suppressed by coke, its release is at first enhanced. Only after the body's supply of serotonin is depleted, and further production slowed, does the cocaine user experience an increasingly strong response to cocaine.

The imbalance of neurotransmitters may be responsible for many of the physical withdrawal symptoms experienced by heavy chronic cocaine users who stop taking the drug: depression, paranoia, lethargy, anxiety, insomnia, nausea and vomiting, sweating, and chills. These are symptoms of the body struggling to regain its normal chemical balance of neurotransmitters.

VITAMIN LOSS

In addition to the other body substances with which cocaine plays havoc, researchers know that the drug also leads to severe vitamin deficiencies, resulting in abnormal neuron functioning. A study conducted by Dr. Gold at Fair Oaks Hospital found that fully 73 percent of cocaine-abuse patients had at least one vitamin deficiency, most frequently Vitamin B6. Vitamins B1 and C levels were also frequently low. Amino acid and metal deficiencies as well have been detected among chronic coke users.

The malnutrition common among chronic users may be only a symptom of some more fundamental action of cocaine. "Severe cocaine abusers tend to ignore all bodily needs, including eating," says Dr. Gold. "The question is, *why* are they uninterested in food?" The answer is even now being sought by Dr. Gold. Meanwhile, an important part of his treatment program for cocaine abusers is providing a diet rich in vitamins and minerals, which appears to increase the chance of successfully kicking the drug habit.

BEHAVIORAL AND PHYSIOLOGICAL EFFECTS CORRELATED WITH NEUROTRANSMITTERS

Dopamine (DA)	Norepinephrine (NE)	Epinephrine (E)	Acetylcholine (ACH)	Serotonin (5-HT)
Normal				
Locomotor hyperactivity Anorexia Sexual stimulation	Increased energy Increased assertiveness (Euphoria)	Increased energy mobilization	Increased mental acuity Muscular coordination	Sleep Tranquilization Antidepressant activity
Excess				
Stereotyped activity Hallucinations Suspiciousness	Agitation Restlessness Anxiety	Cardio-respiratory overstimulation leading to failure	Muscle tremor & incoordination Memory problems	Euphoria Mood elevation
Deficiency				
Extra pyramidal symptoms Parkinsonism Depression	Depression Lethargy	Lethargy	Mental confusion Hallucination	Insomnia Depression Agitation

8
EFFECTS ON THE BODY

At one time or another, all cocaine users will experience at least a few of the drug's many effects.

Every individual has a particular set of sensitivities, reactions and perceptions that will influence the cocaine experience. Even the surroundings in which coke is used—among friends, with strangers, alone, at a party—will alter the drug's impact. A user may feel only some of cocaine's most common effects, but not others; in a different setting, a completely alien set of effects might be felt.

Despite what most moderate coke users may believe, the drug's biological effects are virtually identical whether it is snorted, swallowed, smoked, or injected. Subjective differences arise from the speed at which the effects occur, as well as their strength and duration.

Free-base smoking, and using cocaine by injection, produce the quickest and most marked effects—for the shortest time. These methods also pose the greatest immediate health dangers. Cocaine free-basing provides the most effective means for the body to absorb coke: into the lungs, where an enormous supply of blood brings it quickly to the brain. While producing an incomparable "rush," free-basing also puts extraordinary stress on the body.

THE OVERALL PICTURE

Cocaine's psychological and physical effects begin rapidly regardless of the way it is used. The body's peak reaction to the drug occurs about five minutes after it is taken, and declines steadily over the next 5–6 hours. Following an initial euphoria, which may seem to be the strongest part of the cocaine experience because it is so vastly different from the minutes immediately preceding it, the bulk of cocaine's effects takes place between 20 and 40 minutes after use.

The body reacts to the infusion of cocaine by:

- Increasing the heart rate
- Raising blood pressure
- Speeding respiration
- Increasing body temperature
- Raising blood-sugar levels
- Dilating eye pupils
- Increasing urge to urinate, defecate, or belch
- Depressing appetite
- Increasing restlessness
- Altering muscle control.

Following cocaine's stimulation, irritability and depression may set in due to coke's "burn-out" of the body chemicals that keep moods in balance. There is also a drop in blood pressure and heart rate to levels lower than normal.

These "down-side" symptoms often lead the cocaine user to seek another round of stimulation. And then another. Enough repetitions, over a sufficiently long period of time—a month or less for one person, a year or so for another—can lead to chronic cocaine abuse which, in turn, will probably result in physical deterioration.

The malnutrition that often results from extended cocaine use can lead to various kinds of infections, seizures, or periods of loss of consciousness. Injecting cocaine can cause hepatitis or endocarditis, an inflammation of the lining of the heart.

COCAINE AND THE NOSE

There are more than a few jokes in circulation about noses falling off from cocaine use. In reality, they don't. But what *can* happen may feel just as bad, and become increasingly worse the more coke is used.

The cold, numb, or burning nose, palate and tongue known as the cocaine "freeze" is due to coke's powerful action as a topical anesthetic.

Anesthesia of the palate and tongue causes loss of appetite and dry throat, and constriction of blood vessels in the nose prevents normal blood flow. When full blood movement resumes, several serious problems occur, such as

—Congestion, sneezing, and head cold symptoms
—Irritation, inflammation, sneezing, sniffling, and nasal dripping
—Chronic rhinitis (runny, clogged, inflamed, swollen, ulcerated, painfully sensitive, bleeding nose prone to causing sneezing fits)
—Upper respiratory infections, colds, and bronchitis
—Burns and sores caused by undiluted and/or insufficiently chopped cocaine, or by clumping of sugars used for cutting coke
—Septal necrosis, the death of the tissue (septum) separating the nostrils, causing a hole in the tissue. (The condition is much rarer than believed, but requires surgical repair the infamous "Teflon" nose job—when it does occur since the septum helps avert colds and respiratory infections.)

Some users rinse their nasal passages with water or a saline solution after a session with cocaine, to dislodge and wash away remaining particles. A quarter teaspoon of salt is dissolved in a cup of warm water; a small amount is poured over the thumb and forefinger pinched together, and carried to the nose, where the moisture is briskly sniffed so a slight salt spray is inhaled into each nostril.

Vitamin E oil or glycerine can help prevent drying, cracking and bleeding of nasal membranes caused by cocaine. Ointments such as those sold for diaper rash work for infrequent cocaine use. A few drops of the oil are used to moisten a cotton swab; the swab is carefully inserted into each nostril, and gently rubbed against the tender nasal membranes until they have an even, thin coating of the oil.

If bleeding or irritation continues, or if symptoms like a bad cold are not relieved, the cocaine user is wise to immediately seek medical help.

COCAINE'S 3 REACTION PHASES

Most seriously affected by cocaine are the body's respiratory, cardiovascular, and central nervous systems. In a healthy person, all three work together closely to keep the mind and body in synchronization and operating smoothly. When coke is introduced, the drug changes the way each system functions and damages the delicate interplay between these major body systems.

Although the precise effects on breathing, blood circulation, and the brain and nerves depend on such factors as the cocaine dose, the way it was used, and the individual's personal history of cocaine involvement, the drug might cause an evening of euphoria . . . or an emergency trip to the hospital from what is commonly called a "Casey Jones" overdose.

Coke expert Dr. George Gay, of San Francisco's

Haight-Ashbury Free Medical Clinic, says "Casey Jones" is an apt description of the typical overdose emergency. The name stems not only from the legendary train engineer, he explains, but from the song by The Grateful Dead rock group:

"Casey Jones"

Driving that train
High on cocaine
Casey Jones you'd better watch your speed
Trouble ahead
Trouble behind
And you know that notion
Just crossed my mind.*

The genuine "Casey Jones" reaction is a worst-case scenario, troublesome to emergency-room physicians not only because of its deadly nature, but also because its early symptoms are so similar to a milder, nonfatal coke overdose. In the more serious emergencies, all three major body systems experience severe reactions in rapid progression, resulting in convulsions within as little as two to three minutes, and usually ending in death.

There are less severe reactions to cocaine, of course, which can lead—at least initially—only to some degree of discomfort. Physicians prefer to divide the results of cocaine consumption into three phases. Phase I includes most of the symptoms sought by those using cocaine, such as euphoria, and many less appealing ones, such as tremors and cold sweats, that, while not particularly dangerous, are incredibly uncomfortable.

Anyone experiencing Phase II symptoms, or who says he feels "wrong" or is worried about collapsing, MUST BE TAKEN TO A HOSPITAL EMERGENCY ROOM IMMEDIATELY, since such serious symptoms as these are potentially life-threatening.

*Music by Jerry Garcia; words by Robert Hunter. © 1970 Ice Nine Publishing Company. Used with permission.

Phase III—the central nervous system's part of the "Casey Jones" reaction—can end in death if more than a few symptoms are present, or if they are joined by equally severe symptoms in other major body systems.

COCAINE AND THE NERVOUS SYSTEM

Phase I Nervous System Reactions

Phase I responses of the central nervous system to cocaine are considered mild to moderate. They are seldom life-threatening, but are often extremely unpleasant to the coke user.

- Euphoria; feeling of soaring, well-being; sense of being on top of the world
- Elation; expansive good humor; laughing, or an introverted, withdrawn elation
- Talkativeness; garrulousness
- Excitement; emotional instability
- Restlessness; irritability; apprehension
- Inability to sit still
- Scratching and picking at the skin
- Grinding teeth
- Nausea; vomiting; vertigo
- Sudden headaches
- Cold sweats
- Tremors
- Twitching of small muscles, especially of the face, feet, and fingers
- Tics
- Jerking
- Temperature rise
- Talking about impending doom
- Limited hallucinations ("snow lights," coke "bugs," other hearing, smelling, or tasting hallucinations)
- Psychosis resembling paranoid schizophrenia.

Phase II Nervous System Reactions

Anyone exhibiting Phase II reactions to cocaine SHOULD BE TAKEN IMMEDIATELY TO A HOSPITAL EMERGENCY ROOM, because these symptoms are quite possibly life-threatening, and treatment is best left to professionals.

- No response to voices or other stimuli
- Reflexes of deep tendons greatly increased
- Increased flexibility of limbs and body
- Convulsions
- Epileptic seizures
- Inability to control urine and bowel movements.

Phase III Nervous System Reactions

Phase III reactions of the central nervous system to cocaine pose THE DANGER OF RAPID DEATH to anyone experiencing them. ANYONE WITH THESE SYMPTOMS MUST RECEIVE IMMEDIATE EMERGENCY MEDICAL ATTENTION. (See "Emergency First Aid," Chapter 12.)

- Flaccid muscle paralysis
- Coma
- Fixed and dilated pupils
- Loss of reflexes.

COCAINE AND THE RESPIRATORY SYSTEM

The respiratory reactions which strike cocaine users are caused by the excessive stimulation to the central nervous system and by the irritation to the lungs and throat of breathing cocaine-laden smoke during free-basing.

Phase I Respiratory Reactions

As with cocaine's effects on the other major body systems, there are three distinct phases of respiratory symptoms caused by coke. Phase I respiratory reactions are comprised of mild to moderate symptoms which, while uncomfortable, are not considered especially dangerous.

- Increased breathing rate
- Deeper breathing
- Difficult breathing.

Phase II Respiratory Reactions

Phase II breathing responses to cocaine are extremely dangerous, requiring emergency medical attention. ANYONE SUFFERING FROM THESE SYMPTOMS SHOULD BE RUSHED TO A HOSPITAL EMERGENCY ROOM IMMEDIATELY.

- Gasping, rapid, and/or irregular breathing known as Cheyne-Stokes breathing
- Lack of oxygen.

Phase III Respiratory Reactions

Any breathing symptoms in this category require IMMEDIATE EMERGENCY MEDICAL ATTENTION, since they are POTENTIALLY LIFE-THREATENING. (See "Emergency First Aid," Chapter 12.)

- Total breathing failure
- Accumulation of fluids in the lungs
- So-called "death rattle," gasps of agony just before death.

Free-Basing and the Lungs

Chronic free-base smokers, beyond the danger of injury through explosion of volatile chemicals or death by overdose, face several symptoms common to tobacco smokers, among them:

- Tracheitis and bronchitis, as the lining of the respiratory tract is severely damaged
- Hoarseness, and loss of voice in severe cases
- Coarse, heavy, moist coughs, and wheezes over upper and middle parts of lungs
- Coughs producing mucus and pus, and sometimes blood, and even tarry free-base compounds which have been incompletely burned.

COCAINE AND THE CARDIOVASCULAR SYSTEM

Most cocaine users will experience only those cardiovascular symptoms outlined below in Phase I, which are considered coke's mild to moderate effects. Phase II and III symptoms are much more serious, requiring professional medical attention. Taking cocaine by injection is particularly dangerous to the cardiovascular system, as it can bring about a collapse of blood vessels. Free-basing is the method of use most often leading to heart attacks.

Phase I Cardiovascular Reactions

- Pulse rates increase by 30–50 percent
- Blood pressure increase of 15–20 percent
- Irregular heartbeat
- Pounding heart
- Pale skin due to loss of adequate blood flow.

Phase II Cardiovascular Reactions

Anyone experiencing the cardiovascular reactions to cocaine listed here MUST BE RUSHED TO A HOSPITAL EMERGENCY WARD IMMEDIATELY.

- Ventricular contractions
- Extremely high heart rate and blood pressure, possibly resulting in hemorrhage or congestive heart failure
- Rapid falls in blood pressure and irregular heartbeats, with inadequate blood flow
- Rapid, weak, and irregular pulse
- Skin turns bluish from lack of oxygenated blood supply.

Phase III Cardiovascular Reactions

These symptoms pose THE DANGER OF RAPID DEATH. Anyone experiencing one of these cardiovascular reactions to cocaine MUST RECEIVE IMMEDIATE EMERGENCY MEDICAL ATTENTION.

- Ventricular fibrillation, irregularities of nerve impulses governing heartbeat
- Overall failure of circulation
- Skin turns ashen gray
- Pulse undetectable
- Heart attack
- Heart stops beating.

9
COKE AND THE MIND

An individual's response to cocaine cannot be easily divided into separate "body" and "mind" reactions, since the drug's impact on the cardiovascular, respiratory, and central nervous systems can directly result in changes of mood and emotion.

When a "toot" of cocaine suppresses the appetite, for instance, the very absence of a desire to eat can itself alter an individual's emotional outlook. Similarly, other of coke's less dangerous but annoying effects, like a constantly runny nose—experienced by many coke snorters—could affect *anyone's* attitude toward life.

The "mental" effects of cocaine, however, are generally viewed as those involving mood, outlook, and the feeling of euphoria caused by coke. Together with these *subjective* effects, researchers usually tie *objective* responses like clear changes in behavior—a compulsion to constantly clean the living room, for instance—or gross neglect of everyday personal cleanliness.

Since these kinds of behavioral changes are not known to be caused by any of the drug's distinct physical effects (elevated blood pressure cannot be directly blamed for someone's desire to polish a coffee table) but are instead due to the impact of cocaine on emotion and mood, they are generally considered part of coke's mental effects.

Of course, even a person's emotional state, or outlook on life, might have a purely physical cause. One (or more) of the countless subtle alterations that cocaine causes in the brain's chemical balance or electrical fields may, with more research, turn out to be *the* cause of a specific compulsion, such as the "need" to urinate frequently.

It is conceivable that an individual's response to cocaine may, in fact, be due to the drug's specific effects on the unique chemical and electrical properties of that one person's brain, and nobody else's. This would explain why cocaine will make one partygoer become extremely talkative but turn another inward, to quietly contemplate the beauty of a painting, the perfection of a billiard ball, or the next day's full schedule at the office.

Overall health, weight, metabolism, physical strength, attitudes toward the surroundings—even the way users interpret their other reactions to cocaine—all have an impact on their response to coke, which can be different each and every time the drug is taken. Perhaps such varying aspects of each individual's body and mind create an ever-changing balance of chemicals and electrical impulses which, in turn, are affected in a unique way whenever cocaine enters the body.

Little is known today of the relationship between the chemistry of the brain and the particular emotions influenced by cocaine. Dr. Mark Gold says an individual's attraction or aversion to coke "may depend on his or her brain chemistry responsible for regulating that person's normal state of excitation."

A person with "an average or especially low level of excitation" in everyday life, he proposes, "would enjoy the effects, would be euphoric from alertness, energy and overall stimulation." But the individual who is normally "hyperexcited," says Dr. Gold, "may feel uncomfortable" with cocaine's effects "and even develop paranoia from cocaine."

CHASING THE HIGH

The careening moods, delusions of ability, loss of mental functions, distortions of perception, all comprise a brief psychological picture of a cocaine "high," from the perspective of outside observers.

But the coke user himself will insist he's perfectly okay, in complete control, on top of the world, functioning better than ever.

Said one cocaine user to a *Time* reporter: "The cocaine high is the way you feel if you did something with your life. You think, 'For the first time in a long time, I've really got myself together.'"

The primary effects sought by cocaine users are the most fleeting ones: the feeling of rapture, exhilaration, confidence and well-being, sexual excitement. In short, a touch of nirvana.

High-grade coke, if it can be found, delivers this for fifteen minutes or so. But cocaine also delivers a good many other effects that users would rather avoid. Unfortunately, they can't choose which effects to feel and which to skip. So after the euphoria comes the depression. And to escape the depression comes the desire to snort, or shoot up, or free-base yet again.

Another depression begins; another round of cocaine.

The intensity of a person's "high" depends on the amount of cocaine reaching the brain. Contrary to popular belief, the degree of exhilaration is not directly related to the way cocaine is used—whether by snorting or shooting up, free-basing or "chasing the dragon"—except that some methods get more coke to the brain faster than other methods.

When the "high" is reached, its commonly occurring mental effects, both good and bad, include:

Euphoria: The most sought-after (and talked about) response to coke. At low doses (anywhere from one to seven "lines" if snorted, depending on the drug's purity) it has been described as rapture, exhilaration, joy, giddiness, and an intense "rush." At continued high doses (four to nine "lines" depending on purity), agitation and nervous excitability are often reported, sometimes, with chronic abuse, leading to delirium.

Talkativeness: The feeling of rapport with others, with conversation seemingly very easy. At low doses this may be true. At higher doses, however, while the user might feel communication is improved, others are likely to disagree. Controlled experiments have shown that, while the cocaine user believes his conversation is coherent and understandable, those forced to listen seldom understand what is being said, since the user frequently fails to complete sentences, and often omits words crucial to expressing his meaning.

Contentment: A sense of overall happiness and peace. It may be appealing at low cocaine doses, but at high doses it may turn into intense anxiety.

Alertness: A feeling of clarity, speed of thought, and heightened perception. Research confirms that at low doses, cocaine almost always provides apparent raised alertness. Increased concentration may also be common, experts agree, but only when directed to intellectually simple subjects. A sense of improved creativity is no more than a feeling, says Dr. Gold. "There is no evidence that individuals gain deeper supernatural ability or greater knowledge" while using cocaine, his research indicates. "Their omnipotence is only illusional."

Writers and artists who use cocaine, but hope their works will be appreciated by editors, critics, and the general public, reportedly avoid the drug while working. Under coke's influence, they experience "flights of ideas," half-finished thoughts, disrupted associations, and an overall inability to keep track of what's going on in their minds. They know such confusion will show up in their work, making it unusable. Sustained cocaine use results in indecisiveness and memory disturbances, equally destructive to the creative process.

Need for less sleep: A sense of having incredible energy. At low to moderate cocaine doses, this feeling may be attractive, especially for late-night (or all-night) partying. At higher doses, the feeling turns to the discomfort of insomnia.

Heightened self-awareness: The feeling of being closely "in touch" with one's own feelings. The self-awareness at high cocaine doses turns to paranoia.

Altered sexual feelings: Improved sexual prowess and responsiveness reportedly are perceived. Research shows that at low doses coke can, indeed, enhance performance, delay orgasm, and heighten pleasure. Myths abound about the vast power of cocaine to propel men and women alike to remarkable sexual feats and incredible endurance. At high doses, or with chronic use, the picture changes dramatically; cocaine seems to replace the need or desire for sex.

When injected, cocaine has been reported to sometimes produce spontaneous orgasms without direct genital stimulation. Coke "beats sex all to hell," says one user. Eventually, impotence and frigidity result, and even cocaine cannot provide sexual pleasure.

Humor: Reduces appreciation of jokes and desire to laugh. Sense of humor decreases as cocaine dosage increases. "It's the biggest sense-of-humor dampener I've ever seen," reports one user. "Somebody pulls out some cocaine, everybody starts to talk . . . but the smiles go away."

Physical neglect: Poor personal hygiene. As a coke user's obsession with the drug increases, less attention is paid to basic personal cleanliness. Red eyes, bad breath, sloppy dressing, and the constant need for a shower to wash off dried sweat can be outward signs of an individual's heavy cocaine involvement. Neglect of one's surroundings also commonly occurs.

Even physicians—trained to view cleanliness as extremely important—have been known to neglect their own bodies and homes while using cocaine. A *Time* cover story described one cocaine-using doctor this way:

"His skin was covered with sores from malnutrition. The free-basing also caused rashes and made his tongue so swollen that he could barely talk. In one of the fits of rage that accompanied the 'down' periods, he snapped off two teeth. [In his apartment] shards of broken glass pipes formed a thigh-high pile. The apartment was rancid, filled with unwashed clothes and dishes. The doctor did not notice."

Perceptual changes: Hallucinations, distortions, paranoia. Imagining colors are brighter than they once were is a common reaction to coke. Distant objects may appear to be close. Footsteps may be "heard" when there's nobody nearby. Imaginary "coke bugs" might cause itching, discomfort, and horror. A feeling of "electricity" coursing through the body, the sense that arms and legs have grown longer, a feeling of lightness, "out-of-body" experiences, or a sense of

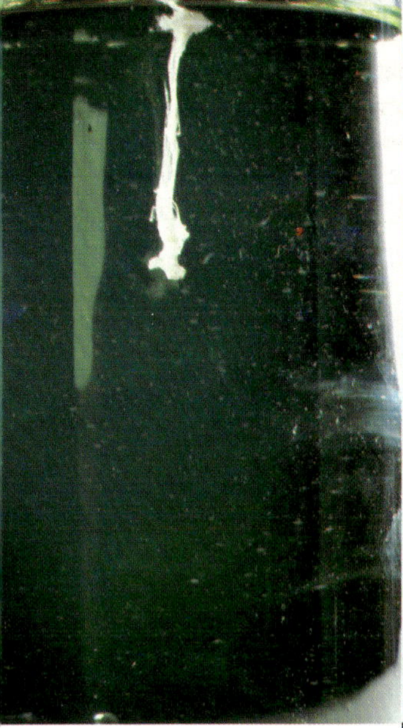

A. COCAINE HCL / 8 SEC.

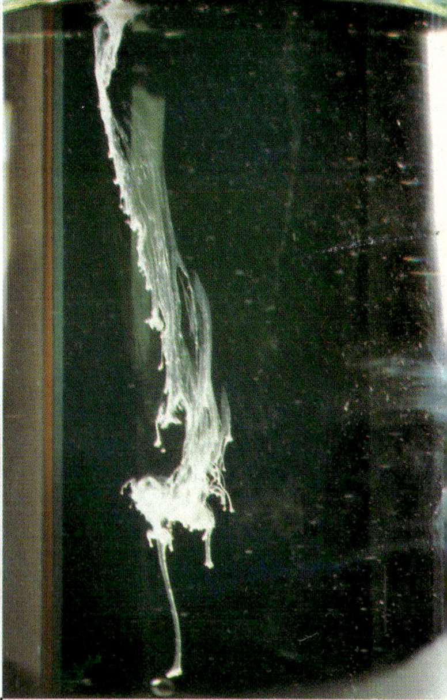

B. COCAINE HCL / 18 SEC.

C. COCAINE HCL / 31 SEC.

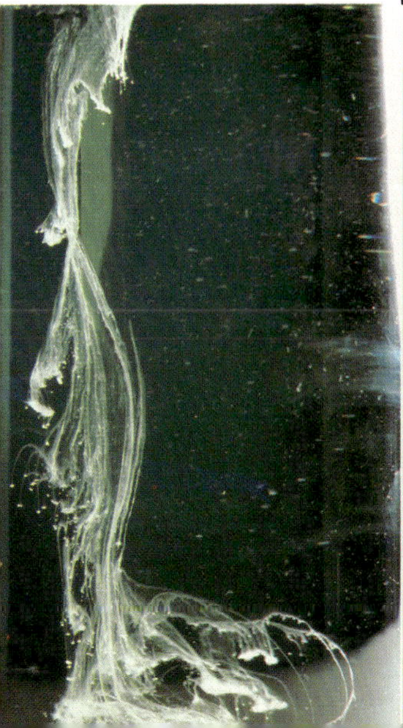

D. COCAINE HCL / 48 SEC.

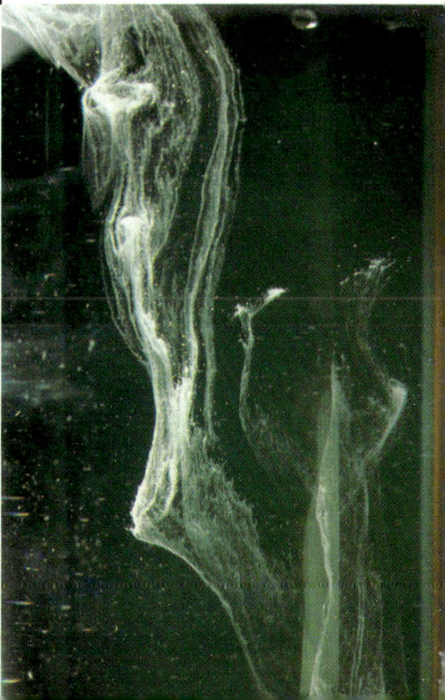

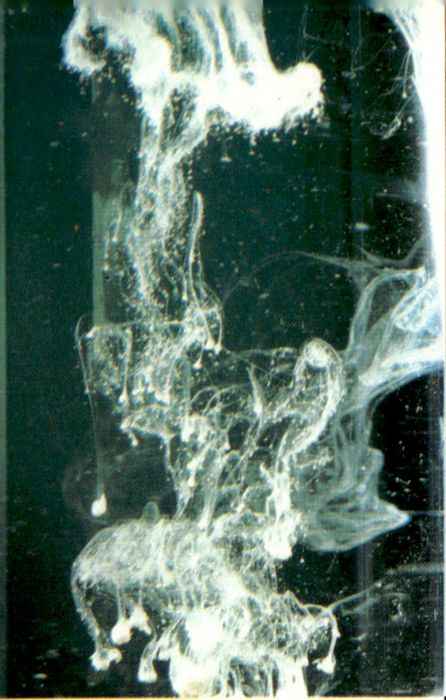

E. “SYNTH COKE” / 4 SEC.

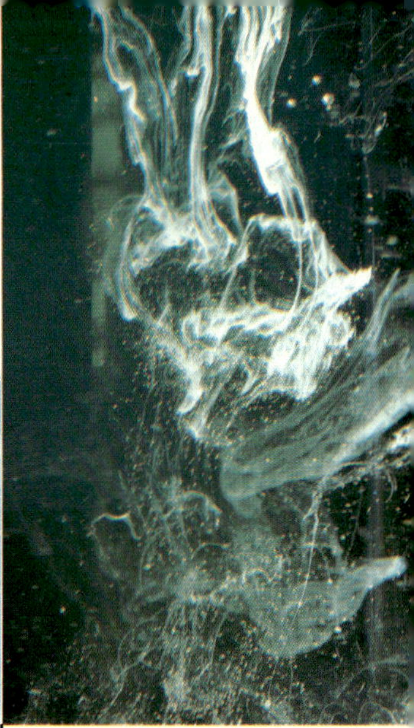

F. “SYNTH COKE” / 13 SEC.

I. LACTOSE / 3 SEC.

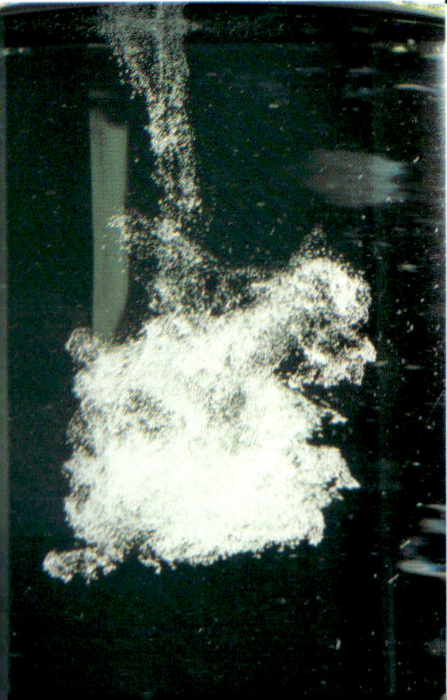

J. LACTOSE / 6 SEC.

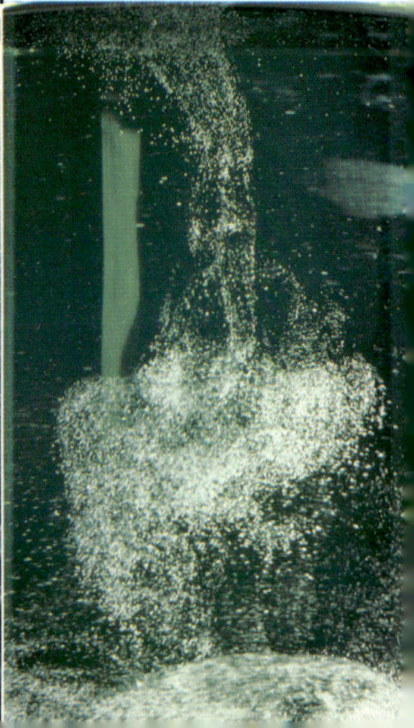

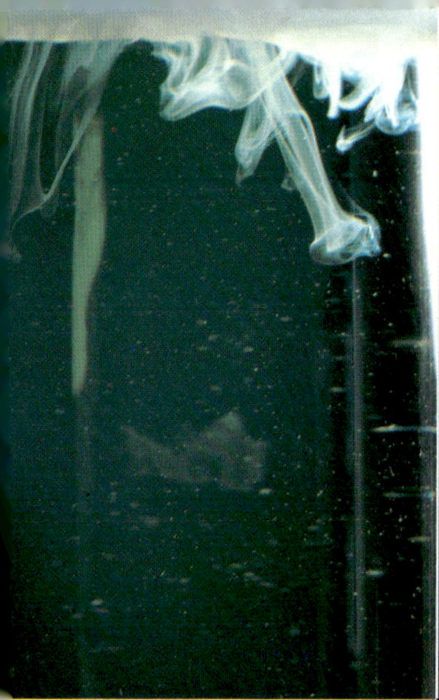

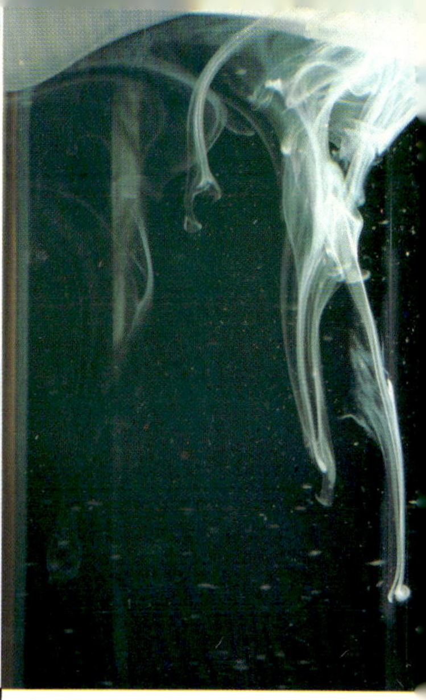

G. D-AMPHETAMINE / 22 SEC.

H. D-AMPHETAMINE / 52 SEC.

K. MANNITOL / 3 SEC.

L. MANNITOL / 9 SEC.

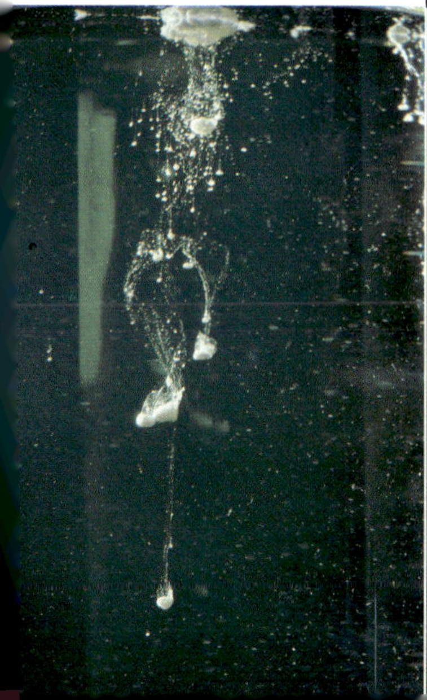

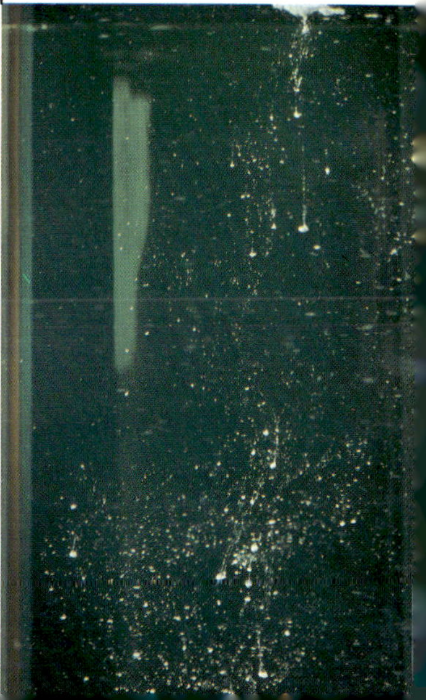

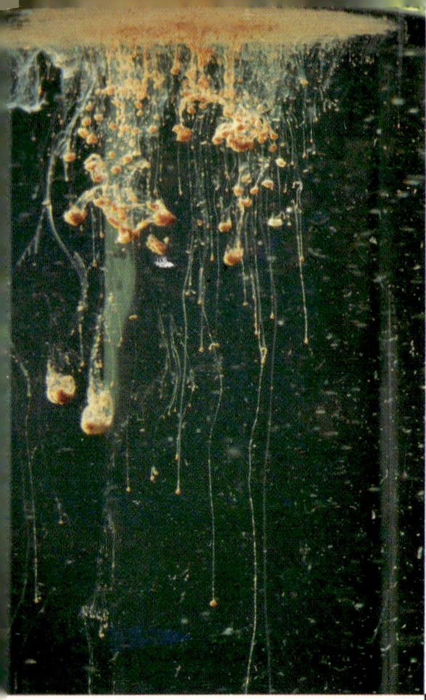

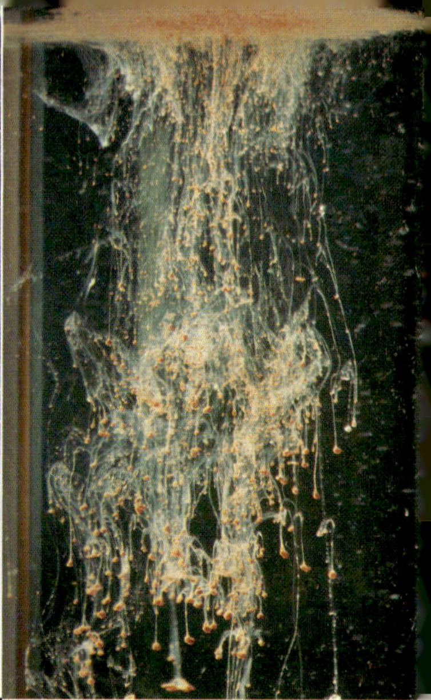

M. "ROCK CRYSTAL" / 10 SEC.

N. "ROCK CRYSTAL" / 15 SEC.

O. "PSEUDOCAINE" / 1 SEC.

P. "PSEUDOCAINE" / 5 SEC.

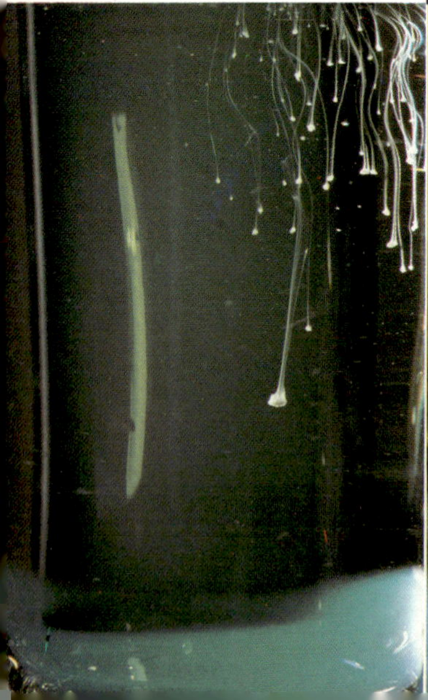

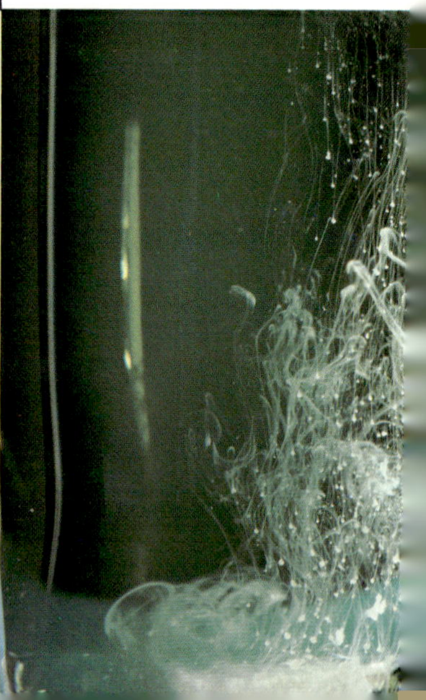

flying, all are perceptual changes which can be caused by cocaine.

Compulsive behavior: Repetitive, stereotyped behavior. Grinding the teeth and constantly chewing are two common behavior patterns among cocaine users. Constant straightening up or cleaning—the stove, the floor, a desk top—is also frequently observed. The user becomes totally absorbed in an apparently meaningless activity.

10
WHAT TO EXPECT

Cocaine can aggravate existing medical problems, and can create completely new ones—many of them serious, even deadly. This list of cocaine's potentially dangerous effects, while extensive, can hardly be complete, since every individual using the drug may respond to it in a unique way. Furthermore, some of these effects may be felt intensely by one user, but barely noticed by another.

GENERAL WARNINGS ABOUT COCAINE

Pregnancy and Nursing: Cocaine, like many other drugs, should be avoided completely by pregnant and nursing women. Since using the drug so often leads to inadequate nutrition, a fetus is likely to receive too little nourishment for proper development. Similarly, the breast milk of a coke user will probably contain too few of the vitamins, minerals, and other substances vital to a nursing infant.

Colds: Snorting coke can lead to continuous symptoms which mimic a bad cold—sniffling, runny nose, etc.—so the user cannot be sure when he really *does* have a cold or the flu.

Bronchitis and Upper Respiratory Infections: Constant irritation of the respiratory tract among free-basers and, to a lesser extent, coke snorters, puts the respiratory system at increased risk for the invasion of bacteria and viruses.

Asthma: Shortness of breath and general breathing difficulties caused by free-basing and snorting, together with anxiety reactions to the drug, can trigger asthma attacks.

Sleep Disorders: Including insomnia and reduced REM sleep. The body can sustain itself just so long without adequate sleep. Prolonged sleeplessness weakens the body. Because cocaine reduces the desire to sleep, frequent users face an overall reduction in the ability to ward off virtually any illness.

Sexual Problems: While coke in small doses may enhance sexual pleasure, larger doses and chronic use can reduce or eliminate sexual desire and ability.

Anxiety: Generalized fears can escalate to the point where hospitalization is required.

Reactions to Environment: Cocaine can trigger exaggerated reactions to the user's surroundings, which can be dangerous if the environment is uncomfortable or unpleasant.

Depression: The more intense the cocaine "high," the deeper will be the depression afterwards.

Addiction: Coke users who are "dependence-prone" can become addicted to the drug, as can almost anyone after extended use (see Chapter 13).

High Blood Pressure: The drug raises blood pressure considerably. Hypertensive users face an increased risk of heart attacks and strokes.

Circulation Problems: Cocaine users who already have poor blood circulation will see their problem grow more severe because of coke's ability to constrict blood vessels.

Heart Problems: Angina pectoris, strong chest pains due to a poor blood flow to the heart, is compounded by cocaine.

Epilepsy or Predisposition to Seizures: Seizures and convulsions can be caused by cocaine. Those with epilepsy, or a predisposition to seizures, confront a greater danger with coke.

Diabetics: Cocaine increases blood-sugar levels, a special danger to diabetics.

Low-dose Overdose: A limited number of people cannot properly metabolize cocaine, which permits even a tiny dosage to remain in the body much longer than usual. A history of breathing problems caused by general anesthesia during surgery or by the use of the muscle relaxant Anectine indicates the potential for a cocaine "overdose" after limited coke use.

COCAINE SIDE EFFECTS

The side effects of cocaine are commonly considered to be temporary, and generally harmless. Some, however, can cause intense discomfort. And, among people with existing medical problems, they can be very dangerous. *A few side effects are identical to signs of a cocaine overdose; anyone exhibiting these should be watched closely for other overdose signals.*

- Rapid pulse rate
- Elevated blood pressure
- Increased breathing rate
- Elevated blood-sugar levels
- Sweating
- Raised body temperature
- Nausea, vomiting, abdominal pain (may be signs of overdose)
- Constriction of blood vessels at point where cocaine contacts tissue (particularly dangerous if drug is applied to sex organs)
- Dry mouth (chalky feeling)

- Dilated pupils (may be sign of overdose)
- Headache (may be sign of overdose)
- Tightened muscles, including those controlling bowel movements
- Urge to defecate, urinate, and belch
- Slowdown of digestion and loss of appetite
- Vitamin, mineral, and amino acid deficiency after continued cocaine use.

SERIOUS ADVERSE EFFECTS

Chronic cocaine usage often leads to one or more serious adverse effects, most requiring medical attention, and some of them potentially life-threatening.

Septal necrosis: The death of tissue separating the nostrils (the septum) takes place only after long-term coke snorting without adequate safeguards (washing the nose, etc.).

Severe digestive disorders: Erratic eating patterns and inadequate nutrition can result in chronic digestive problems.

Dehydration: With loss of appetite comes loss of thirst, which can severely dehydrate the body.

Anorexia and significant weight loss: Permanent damage to various body systems, and lowered resistance to disease, result from cocaine's appetite-suppressant property. Death can occur from the effects of malnutrition.

Loss of sexual desire/ability: Cocaine becomes more important than sex with continued high doses.

Hallucinations: Auditory and visual hallucinations usually accompany chronic use of cocaine, and may be signs of an overdose.

Abscesses, swelling, and blood clots: Injecting cocaine can result in all the adverse effects of shooting up common among heroin addicts. Most dangerous are blood clots which can travel through the circulatory system and cause pulmonary embolisms, strokes, or heart attacks.

Psychosis and paranoia: Delusions so serious that hospitalization is required.

Addiction and compulsive use: Finding and using cocaine become a person's sole concerns in life, until treatment is sought or death occurs.

Multiple drug abuse: In the search for additional stimulation, or relief from post-cocaine depression, other drugs become part of the coke user's repertoire.

Critical cardiac problems: Arrhythmias, heart attacks, and other potentially deadly cardiac conditions can result from coke abuse, especially among those with existing heart or circulatory problems.

Seizures and convulsions: Particularly dangerous to epileptics, these can also strike people with no history of seizures, and may rapidly lead to death.

11
USUAL DOSE AND TOXIC DOSE

The usual dose of cocaine varies according to the method of taking the drug, and the degree of each individual's experience with coke. The dosages described here do not imply that there are safe levels of cocaine, since a dose considered adequate to create a "high" for one person could be deadly for another.

DOSE WHEN SNORTING COKE

A narrow (approximately one-eighth-inch wide) "line" of finely chopped cocaine, two or three inches long, contains between 3 and 30 milligrams, which is usually only between 15 and 50 percent pure coke. One gram of cocaine bought on the street will generally provide 30 to 50 lines. A line is sniffed into each nostril to provide from 20 to 40 minutes of stimulation. A "coke spoon," providing one sniff to each nostril, is usually slightly less than a line.

DOSE WHEN SHOOTING COKE

When injected, either into a vein or beneath the skin, the usual dose is between 8 and 16 milligrams of cocaine. Shooting cocaine produces a faster, more intense "rush" of stimulation than snorting, but the effect is not as long-lasting. Thus far, the greatest number of cocaine deaths result from this method. Shooting up on cocaine sometimes causes rapid death even when the actual dose is less than a dosage considered safe for another method.

DOSE WHEN FREE-BASING

A free-base "hit" can equal about one-fifteenth of a gram (it is sometimes called a "fifteenth"), or about 67 milligrams, or it can be a "tenth," equal to about 100 milligrams. Free-base smokers may take as much as 30 grams in a 24-hour period.

COCAINE'S TOXIC DOSE

Dozens of factors contribute to determining a cocaine dose that would be toxic to a specific person. The extent of previous usage, personal reactions to the drug, and the presence of other drugs in the body can all have an impact on the toxic dose. In general, snorting a "line" of coke every ten to twenty minutes will add up to a dosage of one to four grams daily. In most people this is sufficient to produce behavior changes, psychosis, and other symptoms of toxicity described in Chapter 8.

OVERDOSE LEVELS

In 1977 the American Medical Association suggested that the maximum safe dose of cocaine, when clinically administered, is 200 milligrams per 70 kilograms (155 pounds) of a person's weight, or 3.5 milligrams per kilogram (2.2 pounds) of weight, every 30 minutes. Death can occur even at such low dose levels, and even lower levels if street cocaine is cut with substances to which the user is especially sensitive. There is no "safe" dosage of street cocaine. Users should be alert for the reaction phases described in Chapter 7, which may require emergency medical treatment.

Medical texts state that an initial safe dose is 3 milligrams per kilogram of body weight, an even more conservative figure.

Experts agree a single fatal dose of pure cocaine is somewhere between 1.2 and 1.4 grams taken orally by an individual weighing 150 pounds; or 750–800 milligrams if injected. There is a real danger of overdose from *any* amount of free-base use. A healthy human body is probably capable of metabolizing (and thus detoxifying) the above mentioned amount of cocaine every hour, so it is possible—but barely so—for someone to survive repeated near-deadly doses.

12
EMERGENCY FIRST AID FOR COCAINE OVERDOSE

Magic medicines or secret cures are not available for a cocaine overdose.

The unpleasant fact is that a large percentage of overdose victims die within a few minutes, or on their way to a hospital. Those who survive probably never forget the emergency room experience: breathing tubes stuffed down their throats, countless needles jammed through their skin, day after endless day of poking, prodding, and testing their urine, blood, breathing, and heartbeat.

Outside a hospital, there is little anyone can do about an overdose. But this brief list of ABSOLUTE REQUIREMENTS may one day save your life, or the life of someone you love.

ESSENTIAL EMERGENCY STEPS

1. **STAY CALM.** If you suspect a cocaine overdose (or an overdose of *any* drug), try not to panic. Breathe deeply a few seconds, collect yourself, and decide logically what you should do first.

2. **KNOW THE SYMPTOMS.** Typical cocaine overdose symptoms include lightheadedness, delirium, drunk-like reactions, breathing difficulties, convulsions and uncontrolled muscle spasms, and unconsciousness. A peculiar and deadly breathing pattern known as "Cheyne-Stokes" breathing might occur: the victim takes deeper and deeper breaths, then increasingly shallow breaths for a time, with brief periods of no noticeable breathing mixed in. Breathing may stop altogether, and the heart may stop beating. (See Chapter 10 for more detailed overdose information.)

3. PERFORM ARTIFICIAL RESPIRATION. The most important thing you can do is help the overdose victim breathe, and, if you know cardiopulmonary resuscitation, keep the victim's heart working as well. It's not difficult to perform mouth-to-mouth resuscitation. Make sure the victim's throat is not blocked, pinch the nose shut, take a deep breath, and exhale into the person's mouth. Keep it up!

4. CALL FOR HELP. While continuing mouth-to-mouth artificial respiration as much as possible, grab a phone (drag the unconscious victim with you if necessary) and call for help. If possible, call the emergency number for your area, police or fire department, or poison control center. Explain the emergency and follow instructions exactly.

5. GO TO THE HOSPITAL. If there is no chance (and *only* then) that help will arrive soon, take the victim to the nearest hospital emergency room, by car, cab, tractor, or any means possible.

6. BRING A DRUG SAMPLE. Whenever possible, take a small sample of the drug to the hospital with you, or have it transported along with the victim. Cocaine is adulterated with so many substances which could contribute to the danger that a physician may have to carefully analyze the sample to determine what other chemicals are involved.

7. DO NOT GIVE VICTIM ANY DRUGS, even if you think they might help. There is no antidote to a cocaine overdose, except extraordinary medical care by trained professionals.

13
DEPENDENCE AND ADDICTION

THE '80s ADDICT

Until a few short years ago, the classic definition of a drug addict combined two myths. An addict was thought to be a poverty-stricken, pitiful wreck, writhing in physical and mental agony, stealing, mugging, and terrorizing society in search of his "junk." And the addict's drug could only be one which caused a dreadful physical response when discontinued, such as heroin. Without these withdrawal symptoms—heavy sweating, intense pain, a desire to die—there was no addiction.

Cocaine enthusiasts keep these historic images of the drug addict in mind—as do others who use psychoactive pills, pot, and booze—to convince themselves that coke is not addictive, and they aren't hooked.

But it is now apparent, to anyone who is willing to look, that a drug need not cause serious withdrawal symptoms to be addictive. In keeping up with the age of cocaine, the definition of an addict has changed. Today, anybody who compulsively uses *any* drug, and continues using it despite adverse consequences to personal, professional, or economic health, is considered to be addicted.

Drug abuse is, today, recognized as something more than a problem affecting the poor or misguided. And experts now agree that drug abuse cannot be written off as a mere moral failure on the part of the abuser. Too many new addicts are not "junkies" in the traditional sense, but are part of the "establishment."

They are leaders, not followers. Wealthy, not poor. Well-educated, not school dropouts. Legitimate business people, not thieves.

Drug addiction is seen today as a disease. As is the case with so many other diseases, drug addiction can strike without warning. And, like other diseases, it can be medically treated.

The first sign of addiction to cocaine, or to any drug, for that matter, is *dependence*. A user begins to rely on the drug to get through the week, to survive another day, to last one more hour. Without the drug, everyday life is unbearable; with it, life can be enjoyed—that's dependence.

Increased *tolerance* to the drug is the next step toward addiction. The same dose no longer has the desired effect. One or two "lines" of coke don't seem to provide the same "rush"; it now takes three or four, then six or seven—that's tolerance.

Drug *addiction* often follows a growing dependence and increased tolerance. For decades, addiction has been defined by the body's reaction when a drug is withdrawn. Severe headaches, nausea, or tremors a day or so after the last dose, for example, would demonstrate addiction. A vague longing for the drug would not. The definition has broadened considerably in recent years to include any serious symptom, whether physical or psychological, experienced during drug withdrawal. A person giving up cocaine can become depressed, irritable and paranoid—that's addiction.

PREDISPOSED TO ADDICTION

Researchers now know that some people can become dependent on a drug at very low dosages, often no more than a doctor's normal prescription for one or another ailment. These people are among the 10 percent of the population who may have a genetic predisposition to addiction.

Some are prone to alcoholism. Others tend to grow dependent on tranquilizers. Many may begin relying on cocaine after only a few small doses. At present, there is no sure way to tell in advance which individuals possess a genetic tendency toward addiction. But statistically, the knowledge of alcoholism's family pattern offers a clue to addiction chances with other drugs.

Dr. David Smith, whose Haight-Ashbury Free Clinic in San Francisco has conducted extensive research into addiction, reports that when one parent is an alcoholic, the chances of a son or daughter facing alcohol addiction is thirty-five times higher than the general population. If both parents are alcoholics, the likelihood of alcoholism among children increases by a factor of 400.

Even if neither parent is an alcoholic—perhaps alcohol was never used in the family, so the latent genetic trait never surfaced—if someone has a family or personal history of dependence on *any* drug, he is at greater risk of addiction than most people.

Similar statistics are thought to apply to cocaine.

Dependence on a drug can be either physical or psychological. With cocaine, it has long been acknowledged that the drug's risk of creating psychological dependence is very high. Research is just now demonstrating that coke also carries the danger of some physical dependence. In reality, the distinction is less important than it may seem. The brain, after all, is part of the body, and if the consciousness within the brain demands cocaine, the body will act to get the drug.

ANIMAL RESEARCH

Details of some animal research into cocaine addiction:

Monkeys permitted to self-inject cocaine increased their dosages for several weeks until suffering convulsions and dying. Their pattern was to inject the drug around-the-clock for two to five days, recover for up to five days, then begin injections again. They gave up eating, drinking, sleeping, and sex. Not one animal discontinued cocaine on its own.

Rats were allowed to self-inject coke until researchers discontinued the drug. The animals then independently tried getting more cocaine an incredible 2,000–4,000 times *an hour*.

Monkeys worked five times harder to get cocaine than they did for amphetamine. They worked nine times harder to get cocaine than Benzedrine.

Determining the precise level of cocaine's physical dependence is, in any case, extremely difficult. Animal studies, in which primates were provided with an unlimited supply of coke, demonstrate that the drug will be consumed to the almost complete exclusion of anything else. Food is ignored while cocaine is available, and the primate's usual grooming practices are forgotten. When the cocaine is removed, the animals show several symptoms of great unhappiness bordering on utter misery—clearly a withdrawal syndrome.

The most critical aspects of withdrawal, however, are psychological, the so-called "cocaine blues," during which lassitude, lethargy, irritability, fear, and nervous discomfort with vague "needs," "urgings," and "cravings," are joined by paranoia. Excessive sleeping (hypersomnia) and excessive eating (hyperphasia) also occur. The only "cure," from the user's viewpoint, is more cocaine.

"At first I started using [cocaine] for a crutch for everyday activity," recalls one former coke addict, "the way some people reach for a cup of coffee, to stay awake. Then I got to where I felt I could function better with it. Then I got to where I thought I *couldn't* function *without* it."

"I'M NOT ADDICTED!"

Another key component of dependence and addiction is *denial*. Most cocaine addicts—and abusers of other drugs—refuse to acknowledge their dependence.

Some addicts will point out that they have stopped using the dangerous drug; in reality, they have only switched to another equally damaging drug which provides a similar experience. Often they become hooked on both drugs. This "cross-addiction" occurs, for instance, when a cocaine addict stops using coke, turns to amphetamine for a "high," and ends up dependent on both.

Newspaper articles are filled with reports about famous men and women arrested for cocaine possession. "I use coke, but I'm not addicted," many insist. "I can handle the drug." Only later—at a criminal trial or during treatment—does it become clear to them, and their fans, that they were denying their obvious cocaine dependence.

"I've seen guys buy a 50-cent piece ($50 worth of cocaine) in the morning and by 11 A.M. they don't have any and are looking to get some more," says George Hicks, director of the New Well drug program in Newark, N.J. "Yet they'll tell you they don't have a habit."

COCAINE IMPAIRMENT

Beyond causing addiction and leading to the agony of withdrawal, cocaine impairs the user's ability to effectively function in society. One study, sponsored by the National Institute of Drug Abuse, noted that physical problems occur among more than 80 percent of chronic cocaine users. Psychological and societal impairment, by contrast, is encountered by a full 99 percent of heavy cocaine users.

Among the study's key findings are these problems encountered by coke users:

- Absenteeism from work or school
- Increased reprimands from supervisors
- Loss of job
- Loss or suspension of professional license or certification
- Household discord
- Separation or divorce
- Serious legal problems stemming from investigations, arrests, probation, and/or parole
- Increased debts and other financial problems.

The government study showed *no difference* in the level of such problems among users employing different methods of taking cocaine. Even doses as low as one-quarter gram per week resulted in some impairment.

PSYCHOLOGICAL PROBLEMS LINKED TO COCAINE ABUSE

Incidence of cocaine-associated problems among 500 users who called the national 800-COCAINE "Hotline," a telephone advisory service with headquarters at Fair Oaks Hospital, Summit, N.J.

Depression	83%
Anxiety	83%
Irritability	82%
Apathy	66%
Paranoia	65%
Difficulty concentrating	65%
Memory problems	57%
Loss of sex drive	53%
Panic attacks	50%
Attempted suicide	9%

Fair Oaks Hospital, Summit, N.J. (reprinted with permission of Fair Oaks Hospital, Summit, New Jersey)

WHO GETS HOOKED, AND WHO DOESN'T

Clearly, not everyone who uses cocaine becomes addicted. The vast majority of occasional coke users, in fact, seldom encounter serious problems with the drug. A nine-year study of college seniors actually failed to identify more than a few clear-cut differences between drug users and drug-free students.

This study, completed in 1978, showed more students than ever were using cocaine, which ranked second only to marijuana in popularity. But the results also indicated:

- No difference in grades could be seen between users and nonusers.
- Users were just as likely as nonusers to participate in various campus activities.
- Plans for careers appeared the same among drug users and students who abstained from drugs.

Only two aspects of the study showed obvious differences among the college seniors:

- Drug users were more likely to have seen a psychiatrist than nonusers (but only two percent of those who talked to a psychiatrist believed their problems were drug-related).
- Drug users were more likely to be sexually experienced, although the researchers could not find a cause-and-effect relationship between sexual activity and drug use.

Most cocaine users, it appears, are normal, respectable people.

"Don't be surprised," says one user, "if the guy at the desk next to you just scored for the day." He adds: "My co-workers would laugh in your face if you told them I'm a junkie."

The typical cocaine user, according to statistics drawn from the nationwide toll-free 800-COCAINE hotline, is a 30-year-old male, married, with children—a "junior-executive type," says Dr. Mark Gold, who "came to treatment because he was forced to by an employer who threatened to fire him, or a wife who threatened to walk out."

PERSONAL COCAINE-USE INVENTORY

This list of questions can help you decide whether you are addicted to cocaine or have the potential for addiction. There are no "good" or "bad" answers to many of them—only honest answers. But if you find yourself silently answering "yes" to more than a few, you may be addicted or on your way to addiction.

Is Cocaine Affecting You Financially?

- Has spending money on cocaine kept you from buying necessities, such as food or clothing, or from paying the rent or mortgage?
- Do you worry about how you'll pay for the coke you use?
- Have you ever borrowed money to buy cocaine?

Is Cocaine Affecting Your Work?

- Have you ever missed a day's work because of using cocaine?
- Have you ever used cocaine for "fun" or to "help get through the day" while at work?
- Do your co-workers use cocaine and try to get you to join them?
- Have you been worried lately about losing your job because of your use of cocaine?

Do Drugs Get You into Trouble?

- Have you ever driven a car while you've been under the influence of cocaine and/or drugs and/or alcohol?
- Have you ever had an accident or been given a ticket while you were using cocaine and/or drugs and/or alcohol?
- Have you lost a friend or friends because of your use of cocaine?
- Do you lie about your cocaine use? Even to your close friends?
- Do you sometimes argue with people about the way you use cocaine?

What Are Your Reasons for Your Using Cocaine?

- Do you take cocaine to improve your performance on the job, among friends, in bed?

- Do you use cocaine to feel good, self-confident, the center of the universe?
- Do you take cocaine to help you forget your problems?
- Do you sometimes take cocaine before breakfast, perhaps to get the day off to a "good" start?

Do You Miss Cocaine When You Stop Using It?
- When you don't use cocaine for a day, do you feel depressed?
- Do you feel "left out" when you're not using cocaine?
- Do you sometimes feel sick—a headache,upset stomach, etc.—when you stop taking cocaine for a day or longer?

Does Your Use of Cocaine Bother You at Times?
- Have you lost interest in sex—even a little—since you've been using cocaine?
- Have you ever stopped doing cocaine even temporarily, because of an unpleasant physical or mental feeling?
- Have you ever felt sick while taking cocaine but kept on taking it anyway?
- Have you ever tried to cut down your cocaine use?
- Do you sometimes worry that your cocaine use is out of control?
- Have you ever wondered whether you're addicted to cocaine?
- Do you ever feel guilty about taking cocaine?
- Do you have trouble waking up or feel as if you have a hangover the morning after you use cocaine?
- Do you suspect that your use of cocaine has increased over the past few months?
- Do you think about cocaine at least once a day? More often than that?

Is Cocaine Affecting the Way You Think?
- Have you sometimes thought about suicide since you've been using cocaine?
- Do you sometimes accept cocaine without even wondering about its purity when a friend offers it to you?
- Are you unable to remember what happened after you've used cocaine?

- Do you have trouble concentrating when you've taken cocaine?

Note: Adapted from material in *The Little Black Pill Book*, ed. Lawrence D. Chilnick (New York: Bantam Books, 1983).

14
TREATING DEPENDENCE AND ADDICTION

There is no single *best* treatment for cocaine abuse. The specific care provided to each user will depend largely on his or her immediate needs, and the extent of cocaine involvement.

Several widely accepted rules for dealing with cocaine abuse, however, have been developed by the country's most successful rehabilitation centers and drug abuse experts. Treatment can range from the cautious use of drugs to control the depression and anxiety brought on by cocaine withdrawal, to little more than providing quiet, supportive surroundings while an individual recovers from his cocaine experience.

Organized treatment programs, many of them covered by medical insurance, can cost upwards of $12,000 for a three- or four-week stay amid attractive surroundings, under the care of an experienced staff. Many programs, of course, are much less expensive, but the nature of care needed to help kick the cocaine habit requires a large staff, and thus a higher cost than most other drug programs. In some cases, less-than-ethical physicians are charging more than they should, thus taking advantage of the overall high-income status of their patients.

SYMPTOMS AND THEIR TREATMENT

The cocaine abuser with serious symptoms such as acute anxiety, or psychosis, will probably find himself in a hospital eventually, having sought help on his own, or having had the good fortune to be surrounded by friends or family members who cared enough to urge that help be located.

Acute Anxiety

Even at low cocaine doses, sharp attacks of excessive anxiety strike many users. Dr. David E. Smith advises treating cocaine-induced anxiety with a "supportive environment," constant reassurance, and limited doses of a sedative such as diazepam (Valium).

The clinic subscribes to what Dr. Smith calls the "Science of ART" method: "A" standing for "acceptance"; "R" for "reduction of stimulation; rest; and reassurance"; and "T" for "talkdown."

ART TREATMENT

ACCEPTANCE: As the effects of cocaine ebb, staff workers try to impress on the individual that there is no stigma tied to cocaine abuse. Simultaneously, the user is encouraged to regulate his or her own surroundings without the drug.

REDUCTION OF STIMULATION: A quiet, nonthreatening environment is provided, along with a gentle and understanding—but firm—approach by staff members.

TALKDOWN: Talking with the cocaine abuser in a sincere, concerned way about coke and any subject of interest to him or her.

At the San Francisco facility, the ART method is generally carried out in a "quiet room," where outside stimulation, such as radio, television, or newspapers, is prohibited. Individual counseling is mixed with muscle massage to ease spasms. Sedatives are admissible if needed.

Cocaine Psychosis

Psychosis resulting from cocaine abuse is extremely frightening to the user, as well as to others. And it can be deadly. Of more than 100 cocaine-related deaths analyzed in one study, fully 60 percent were either suicides or murders. Cocaine psychosis is characterized by extreme paranoia—uncontrolled suspicions about anything and anybody—as well as hallucinations.

Cocaine psychosis is usually treated with drugs. Repeated small doses of diazepam can be used for sub-psychotic anxiety reactions. Some specialists favor the use of haloperidol or thorazine during hospitalization. If the cocaine psychosis does not diminish, increased doses of those drugs may be used.

Doctors must be alert for indications that an apparent cocaine-induced psychosis may actually be an underlying psychotic condition simply brought to the crisis stage by coke. In such a case, a potent—and more dangerous—phenothiazine-derivative antipsychotic drug may be used.

CHRONIC TOXIC REACTIONS

Because cocaine fosters compulsive use, those able to obtain a large supply will engage in "binges" or "runs" that last until the coke is gone or the user collapses from exhaustion.

Binges of nearly continuous cocaine use can go on for days, or even weeks. But heavy users often face a variety of symptoms, ranging from simply uncomfortable to potentially deadly. They include:

- Hyperactivity
- High blood pressure
- Loss of muscle control (tics, tremors, jerks)
- Distortions of perception
- Delusions.

These symptoms, if not quickly corrected, can lead to life-threatening heart irregularities, strokes, and related ailments. When a cocaine user requires treatment for chronic toxicity, it must take place in a hospital setting and will commonly include:

- Careful monitoring of the blood, respiratory, and nervous systems
- Use of the antihypertensive drug propranolol
- Doses of diazepam.

Drugs like diazepam and propranolol are used to calm the acute anxiety that accompanies cocaine toxicity.

COCAINE OVERDOSE TREATMENT

A cocaine overdose can kill in minutes. Smugglers have died on board commercial airplanes when the cocaine-filled rubber packets (usually condoms or cut-off fingers of surgical gloves) they swallowed to avoid detection burst in their stomachs or intestines, instantly releasing large quantities of coke into their systems.

In one case not long ago, doctors were attempting to remove a swallowed cocaine-filled condom from a smuggler's stomach by using a surgical device to grab hold of the drug cache. The condom burst inside the smuggler during the procedure, and even though he was surrounded by physicians who performed emergency surgery and administered every possibly helpful medication, the smuggler nearly died.

Hospital emergency rooms across the country are reporting more and more cases of overdoses from injected or free-based cocaine.

There are simply no medicines that reduce the drug's deadly effects. Survival depends as much on the ability of the victim's own body to withstand the overdose as on the array of sophisticated equipment available to today's doctors.

A cocaine overdose might cause epilepsy, hyperthermia, dangerously high blood pressure, heart failure, strokes, severe breathing difficulties, and/or severe psychosis. Emergency room physicians deal with dangerous symptoms, not cocaine, although it is important they know what drug is responsible for the overdose. A typical cocaine overdose victim, rushed to the hospital, might receive the following emergency treatment:

- A breathing tube inserted in the throat
- Cardiopulmonary resuscitation
- Intravenous diazepam and/or barbiturates for seizures
- Intravenous muscle relaxants such as succinylcholine, curare, or pancuronium
- Propranolol, a heart drug
- Lidocaine for heart problems
- A rectal thermometer for frequent temperature monitoring
- A cooling blanket, ice water, and/or fans in the event of hyperthermia
- Bicarbonate injections for serious cardiorespiratory problems
- Naloxone in case heroin was also taken
- Sodium nitroprusside, phentolamine, or propranolol

Most victims who reach a well-staffed hospital before they die survive the overdose, although they must sometimes spend weeks in a hospital recovering before they can resume their normal lives.

WITHDRAWAL AND RECOVERY

A number of programs have been created to help cocaine users abstain from the drug once its use becomes destructive or uncontrollable. The Haight-Ashbury Free Medical Clinic recovery plan aims to help the user start conquering depression, anxiety, and lethargy within a week, without medications, although low doses of a sedative are sometimes used.

The Fair Oaks Hospital makes use of tyrosine in battling such withdrawal effects as fearfulness, insomnia, trembling, and nausea, and has also successfully used Naltrexone.

Other researchers have found that the tricyclic antidepressant desipramine can be helpful in cocaine withdrawal, but warn that its potential side effects (heart irregularities among them) should be guarded against.

Withdrawal programs include detailed education on addiction. This is important to the cocaine abuser, who must be made aware that he or she cannot handle the drug *even occasionally* in the future.

Family therapy is an important part of the programs. The support of family and friends will speed the cocaine user's return to normal life. Group therapy with other cocaine abusers is also vital. The type of therapy that made Alcoholics Anonymous a model for recovery from alcoholism works equally well for cocaine abuse. In addition to Cocaine Anonymous and cocaine recovery support groups, individual therapy, in which each cocaine user's unique problems are analyzed, is also incorporated into the recovery programs.

Many heavy cocaine users show signs of severe nutritional deficiencies, and Dr. Mark Gold adds to the other aspects of treatment a diet rich in vitamins, minerals, and amino acids, which he believes greatly enhances the chance of recovery.

Another treatment method in use today is called "contingency contracting," which employs a strong psychological motive to help the user kick cocaine. The idea behind contingency contracting is "If *you* ever use cocaine again, this is what *I* will do!"

As described by Drs. Antoinette Anker and Thomas Crowley of the Department of Psychiatry, University of Colorado, the method works like this: together, the cocaine abuser and a therapist decide on a promised action which will be completed if the abuser uses coke again and which, if completed, will without question greatly embarrass the user or make his or her life even more miserable than would the use of cocaine.

The action might be a signed confession of cocaine abuse and a letter of resignation addressed to the user's boss. Or it might be a large cash contribution to the Democratic Party, even though the coke abuser is a staunch Republican. Whatever the action, it must be of critical importance to the abuser.

The confession, political contribution, or such, is left in the hands of the therapist, who makes a solemn vow to pass it along if cocaine is ever used again.

So powerful is the coke user's need to keep the therapist from forwarding the material that 31 out of 32 cocaine abusers in the Anker-Crowley study remained coke-free using the method. The one individual who returned to cocaine lost his job, but he later entered a residential treatment program and, eventually, signed another contingency contract and now remains drug-free.

WHERE TO FIND HELP

There are now dozens of drug treatment centers with experience in treating cocaine abuse. Appendix C provides a state-by-state address and phone number listing compiled from the extensive resources of the Fair Oaks Hospital.

SELF HELP

Many cocaine abusers try to stop using the drug on their own. Some are successful. Their main strategies:

SELF-CONTROL. By slowly reducing the amount of cocaine used—whether smoked, snorted, or injected—a small handful of men and women have eventually become drug-free. Some began by cutting their coke intake by as much as half every day. Others attempted to stop abruptly (going "cold turkey"). A significant reason for failure is the continuing availability of cocaine; unless no additional supplies are within reach, self-control almost never works for more than a brief period.

SUBSTITUTING OTHER DRUGS. Many of the chemicals used to cut cocaine have effects similar to coke's. Many cocaine users, fearful of coke itself, turn to the other drugs instead. Even tobacco and caffeine are sometimes used as cocaine substitutes. And a large number of coke abusers turn to heroin and other narcotics. Substituting other drugs, though, seldom puts a stop to the cocaine problem; most users tire of the substitutes and return to coke eventually.

SOURCE CONTROL. Some cocaine users deliberately cut their sources of the drug. They ask family members and friends to keep them from buying coke, or to take charge of the money and possessions they might use to purchase it. A few even go so far as to tell cocaine dealers not to sell them any more drugs, and surprisingly, many cocaine dealers honor such requests. But long-range success seems to depend on whether other methods are used at the same time, such as professional counseling.

15
COCAINE: STAR OF STAGE, SCREEN, AND TELEVISION

A prestigious Southern California newspaper explains the etiquette of accepting cocaine at parties . . .

One of TV's most popular entertainers jokes about the West Coast cocaine industry, ending his patter with a fake sneeze typical of chronic coke snorters . . .

A Hollywood luncheon, attended by men and women whose names fill the fashion pages, ends with waiters serving hand-blown glass straws and artfully arranged trays of cocaine . . .

Cocaine—snorted, injected, or smoked—today enjoys almost unbelievable popularity throughout America's entertainment industry. Coke is used by actors and actresses. Singers and dancers. Stand-up comics. Scriptwriters. And an array of men and women who labor behind the scenes to create films, television shows, plays, and commercials.

If the names of stars charged with selling, buying, or possessing cocaine were on a theater marquee for a one-night show, enormous crowds of enthusiastic fans would probably appear.

John Belushi would be unable to join them.

Belushi, whose acclaimed performances on television's *Saturday Night Live* made his name a household word, was hardly the first popular entertainer to lose his life because of drugs. Janis Joplin, Freddie Prinze, Jimi Hendrix, Elvis Presley, and France's "little sparrow," Edith Piaf, are among those who died after being heavily involved with drugs. Nor was Belushi's death, at the age of thirty-three, early in 1982, the first cocaine-related catastrophe to affect a famous entertainer.

Less than two years earlier, in 1980, comedian Richard Pryor was critically burned following seventy-two hours of free-base cocaine smoking. Pryor's injuries were initially attributed to an explosion of highly flammable ether being used to purify coke, but were later explained by the comic himself as due to the accidental ignition of some spilled 151-proof rum. Pryor admitted the accident came hard on the heels of his around-the-clock cocaine binge. After running out of coke, Pryor publicly confirmed, he began drinking the rum he had minutes earlier used to filter cocaine smoke.

The horror of Pryor's accident was graphically described by *Time* magazine (June 23, 1980):

> An explosion rocked his bedroom, and black comedian Richard Pryor was engulfed in flames. Hearing his screams, his maid summoned his aunt Jenny, who rushed to his room and smothered the blaze with bedclothes. In shock, Pryor bolted from the house in the Los Angeles suburb of Northridge and rushed into the street. . . . His polyester shirt had melted onto his arms and chest, and he suffered third-degree burns from the waist up. . . .

The incident focused national attention on the new trend of cocaine free-basing, during which the impure drug is soaked in a strong chemical, like ether, to release the cocaine "base," then slowly smoked through a water pipe often filled with alcohol. (Details about the free-base process are in Chapter 3.)

A subsequent whirlwind of publicity described free-basing as a "dangerous drug craze" and a "hazardous and costly habit." The process of purifying cocaine was carefully described. The availability of legal do-it-yourself kits was pointed out. And the intense pleasure felt by free-base cocaine users was discussed in detail.

The publicity surely forestalled the free-basing of cocaine by some individuals who grew worried about the dangers. But the articles also spurred sales of the very drug paraphernalia—pipes, solvents, etc.—whose use they cautioned against. Although immediately after Pryor was hurt a brief decline in sales was experienced by firms involved in marketing the equipment, the industry recovered almost as fast as did the comedian. Within two weeks, sales of free-base kits had skyrocketed, and some law-enforcement officials blamed the Pryor publicity.

"This exposure amounted to considerable free advertising," reported the *Journal of Psychoactive Drugs*. Even the National Institute of Drug Abuse (NIDA) responded to the publicity by issuing its first official press release on cocaine free-basing, which was, until then, barely recognized as a common means of ingesting the drug.

Simultaneously, journalists trying to describe the free-base process and explain its popularity employed such phrases as "newly fashionable" and "today's trend," as though dangerous free-basing was little different from a display of a new season's styles in a boutique. Drug-abuse experts believe such press coverage served only to enhance the image of cocaine in general, and free-basing in particular.

THE BELUSHI TRAGEDY

Then, on March 5, 1982, another cocaine incident rocked Hollywood's public confidence—there was no longer any question that cocaine was seriously affecting the Hollywood community.

John Belushi, the riotous comedian whose somewhat insane character portrayals on television and in films brought years of laughter to millions of ardent admirers, was found dead of a cocaine-heroin overdose. The combination, known as a "speedball," is generally employed only after a long history of various modes of cocaine use.

A few days after Belushi's death, the *Los Angeles Times,* in a thought-provoking article by Kate Braverman, came to grips with the tragedy and asked several key questions about Tinseltown's emerging cocaine epidemic:

> I imagine his room . . . over-stuffed ashtrays, piles of cocaine and heroin, old room-service trays, empty fifths. . . . It's difficult to turn down the ride when it is yours, effortlessly. When you know the best dope is yours with one phone call. . . . The drugs are always there, even when you don't want them. . . .
>
> You just keep careening wildly out of control, getting richer, finding more acclaim, making people laugh. Would you have the inner strength to stop? Why should you stop? You're in a delirium, the edges have been erased.
>
> It's the American dream. The fat cat laughing, consuming pleasure without border. After all, you're still taking care of business. You're still making those photographic sessions, those inter-

views, another crew is working.

And isn't this what a star does? Isn't that what we pay our stars to do? To explore new terrain, to live larger-than-life sagas . . . ?

Belushi and all too many other stars were drawn to cocaine because of their celebrity status, asserts Dr. Mark Gold.

"Once someone defines himself as a celebrity," Dr. Gold explains, "there is a certain theory of entitlement." The star "figures he is entitled to the best of life, and once he has all that, he figures he's entitled to the best of internal life, by controlling his moods through drugs."

The exhilaration of fame is "more difficult to come by" than the "high" of cocaine, reasons Dr. Gold. And coke quickly becomes the preferred substitute for hard work, which frequently results in only fleeting fame, or none at all.

"Someone like Belushi," says Dr. Milton Greenblatt, professor of psychiatry at the UCLA School of Medicine, "with a special set of talents, claws his way to the top and lands there rather quickly. He doesn't have the maturity, the long history of solid, secure work, enough ups and downs, that he could develop a strong ego so he could take his frustrations with his triumphs.

"For those who reach the heights of their profession at an early age," Dr. Greenblatt continues, "any hiatus between triumphs is trying. It's a risky business for someone to reach these heights too early."

In a somewhat unscientific but nevertheless keen observation, one TV producer explains cocaine's lure in the entertainment industry this way: "There's something in very creative people's genes that make them go to extremes."

ANOTHER COCAINE CASUALTY: DAVID CROSBY

Some famous individuals are badly bitten by the cocaine bug even though their rise to stardom may be significantly slower than Belushi's, and may offer them ample opportunity to get used to the roller-coaster life-style common among entertainers.

David Crosby spent his forty-second birthday looking forward to the start of a five-year jail term for possession of a quarter-gram of cocaine, about $25 worth.

The high-voiced singer of the Crosby, Stills, Nash and Young team—which gained worldwide musical recognition in the '60s and '70s—was manacled and arrested in a back room of a Dallas nightclub, where police found him free-basing cocaine. A .45 automatic was hidden in a bag on his lap.

Crosby had been using cocaine for "several years," claims Hollywood screenwriter Carl Gottlieb, despite the best efforts of his many show-business friends to help him stop. A contingent of well-known entertainers once visited Crosby at his California home urging him to enter a rehabilitation program.

"There was a day or two of reform," remembers Gottlieb, "but then it was over. He was faced with a change of life-style, and he opted out of it."

Prior to Crosby's cocaine addiction, "he was a connoisseur of quality objects," says the screenwriter. "His houses were full of good paintings and art objects he had acquired over the years. I think you can safely say that David has smoked up everything he owned—all the cars, everything."

A Texas judge justified the severity of Crosby's sentencing—possession of such a small amount of cocaine commonly results in a warning or probation—by saying public figures "are more likely to be held up to close scrutiny."

Complained Crosby: "I'm being treated like a murderer."

CALIFORNIA DREAMIN'—JOHN AND MACKENZIE PHILLIPS

There are times, even in the individualistic, ego-oriented world of stage and screen, when more than one member of the same entertainment family is seduced by cocaine or other equally powerful drugs.

Such was the case involving "Papa" John Phillips—whose legendary singing group The Mamas and the Papas blazed like a comet for more than a decade—and his daughter Mackenzie, starlet of the television sitcom *One Day at a Time* and the 1973 movie *American Graffiti*. Their story of cocaine involvement has been recounted in numerous newspaper and magazine articles, and by themselves in public appearances throughout the country.

Mackenzie's brother Jeffrey also used illicit drugs, and a cousin, Patty Throckmorton, died of a heroin overdose at twenty-five. John Phillips' third wife, Genevieve, was another family member who became addicted.

The family's unhappy story has its roots in the free-living '60s. "Papa" John was using marijuana and a pharmacy of psychedelics that were as popular at the time as flower children in San Francisco and anti-Vietnam activism throughout the country.

By the early '70s, he had joined the ranks of Hollywood's cinema and stage celebrities who would snort a little cocaine over cocktails, or pass around some of the magical white crystals at high-flying, weekend-long parties. In those social circles, money was never a barrier to another snort of the expensive drug.

In 1976, the singer-composer—who had already penned such hits as "California Dreamin'" and "Monday, Monday"—flew to London, where he composed the score of David Bowie's film, *The Man Who Fell to Earth*.

A friend, who pushed drugs on the side, moved in with John and his wife for a few weeks, and when he finally moved out, both John Phillips and his wife were hooked on heroin.

When they returned to Manhattan, the couple visited a doctor seeking help to kick their habits. To make heroin withdrawal easier, the uninformed physician told them, they could safely use cocaine.

"Six months later," John says, "we were using cocaine all waking hours. We were so strung out, the only thing that would calm us was heroin or morphine, so we began to go back and forth. Narcotics to come off cocaine, cocaine to come off narcotics."

Visiting a New York pharmacy one day, John spotted some prescription needles. The druggist, thinking he was doing the famous entertainer a favor, offered the syringes as a gift, and continued to provide a steady supply of drugs, including tranquilizers and amphetamines.

Another "friend" provided the forms required by law to purchase potent prescription drugs. The blank documents, which must be filled out in triplicate to satisfy narcotics-control laws when drugs are sold legally through pharmacies, allowed John to buy such a large variety of drugs he cannot recall all their names.

"I had an insatiable cocaine habit," Phillips recalls. "Genevieve and I were doing a quarter-ounce or half-ounce a day. We were also taking 60 Dilaudids a day, 160 milligrams of morphine, heroin, and everything else."

Phillips is convinced that only Elvis Presley, of all the other famous musicians known for their heavy drug use, sampled such variety.

Daughter Mackenzie, meanwhile, was one of Los Angeles' best-known teenyboppers, smoking marijuana and drinking heavily in apparent retaliation for the upside-down life into which she had been thrust.

While still in her early teens, she had become famous for her television performances, and was extremely wealthy. She was also an exceptionally confused young woman. Six schools, a parental split, and money nearly flowing from the faucets led Mackenzie to jail when she was just eighteen. She was charged with disorderly conduct near the Hollywood Strip while under the influence of drugs or alcohol. Those who remember the scene say she was completely out of control when arrested.

A pair of unhappy romances, one of them ending in marriage, soon followed. "I thought I was in love," she recalls, but is now quick to add: "I was stoned. We were all stoned." On coke.

While Mackenzie was busy spending upwards of

$500,000 (!) on cocaine, her father was occupied selling his most valuable possessions to support an astonishingly virulent multi-drug habit. One of the four Rolls-Royces he owned was worth close to $80,000, but to get quick cash for cocaine, he sold it for only $24,000.

John Phillips' life was swirling down the drain faster than his friends thought possible, even considering his heavy drug usage. He started visiting filthy "shooting galleries," decrepit buildings where used needles litter the floors and addicts gather regularly to buy and inject their drugs.

Close friend Mick Jagger, of Rolling Stones fame, would sometimes receive urgent middle-of-the-night phone calls from John's wife, begging Jagger to collect her husband from one shooting gallery or another and bring him safely home. John started having accidents in the cars he hadn't yet sold, and found himself setting fires through carelessness.

Drugs became so all-consuming he simply left a needle in his arm. He was so sure that invisible insects were crawling over his skin that he refused to believe doctors who swore that the uncomfortable sensations were common side effects of the drugs he was taking.

Busted but Grateful

John Phillips was arrested in mid-1980, by federal drug-enforcement agents who raided his Long Island home. Being locked away from drugs "was the best thing that ever happened to me," he would later admit, although his initial fear of punishment, and the agony of withdrawal, must have been terrifying and painful.

While awaiting trial and sentencing—he later served 30 days in a federal prison after being convicted of conspiracy to distribute cocaine—"Papa" John checked into Fair Oaks Hospital in Summit, N.J., for rehabilitation.

Having undergone nearly a dozen prior drying-out episodes, he had no great hopes for success. But the combination of proper diet and exercise, along with a rigidly enforced regimen of drugs like clonidine and Naltrexone—which ease withdrawal symptoms—was something he had not experienced before. The program also included group psychiatric sessions under the direction of Dr. Mark Gold.

The 6-foot, 5-inch singer, whose weight had dropped from 210 pounds to 140 and whose arms were covered with needle scars when he joined the program, had such poor circulation in his hands that they were almost black. As he began to recover from his near-starvation, he gained weight and felt more and more energetic without drugs.

Mackenzie Phillips was at that time languishing in a drug stupor in California. Twice she nearly died of overdoses.

"Basically, I just stayed home shooting cocaine," she later told an interviewer, "sometimes as often as every five or ten minutes. I would leave home only to buy more coke." Mackenzie used cocaine so often, she says, that "I went for days without sleep, stopped eating, ruined my skin, got vitamin deficiencies and anemia, and found that the only way I could get to sleep was by using downers, and even heroin.

"The days and nights just blurred," she says. "I didn't talk about anything but drugs." Like her father, Mackenzie grew extremely thin, ending up a fraction of her former weight at only 90 pounds.

The Phone Call

Mackenzie says she was "finally getting sick and tired of being sick and tired," when she received an unexpected telephone call.

"My father called me from Fair Oaks and asked me to come," she says. "If he hadn't convinced me, I'd either be dead now—or still running."

Of her own treatment, which followed the same course as her father's, she remembers that "psychologically I was totally dependent on cocaine, and it was very hard to come off it. The bad thing about cocaine is that the more you use, the more you become convinced that you *need* it to cope, that you're nothing without the drug."

Since then, Mackenzie returned to *One Day at a Time* (now in reruns) for guest appearances. She and her father have formed a new singing group. Both have committed the bulk of their free time to counseling other drug abusers under treatment in the New Jersey program and elsewhere. They also visit public schools and universities, describing their experiences to groups of students in an attempt to head off future drug disasters.

"Most of the actors and musicians I've known who used drugs ultimately fell apart," Mackenzie says of a host of Hollywood cocaine enthusiasts. "During the time it takes for drugs to ruin a talented person totally, the public gets the impression that the drugs were part of the glamour and the success, [but] if musicians and actors seem to advocate drug use, it's only because they can't get hold of themselves and admit that they're losing it.

"If someone had told me that this could have happened to me," she continues, "I never would have believed it. After all, I had achieved fame, fortune, and success.

"When people offered me drugs, I'd say, 'Oh, just this one time' or 'I really don't have anything to do today.' I'd even fool myself into thinking that I was functioning at work or in life better than before. But it's never just once, and it's never without risk. In the end, drugs nearly destroyed me."

She and her father are still plagued by people, sometimes complete strangers, who offer them drugs in restaurants, hotel lobbies, elevators, and other public places. Says Mackenzie, "We just brush them off. If you handed me a suitcase full of cocaine right now, I'd just laugh and tell you to get out of my way."

Veteran television executive Irv Wilson says of cocaine cases like the Phillipses': "It's hard to stay straight in this business. You have to have a great sense of who you are and what you can do. I've seen cocaine used in offices all over Hollywood. It's become a very socially acceptable thing."

A prominent California psychiatrist says cocaine is an "almost required" part of the "conspicuous consumption out here. We have a lot of people who have a lot of money who buy very exotic, glamorous, high-priced drugs."

This psychiatrist's patients include "a couple of people who are not sure if they really want to quit [cocaine] because it is so mandatory to their positions. They have to dispense it to people they work with. It's almost culturally ingrained in show business, very much like tobacco is ingrained in the armed forces and alcohol is a drug of commerce in much of the business world. Similarly, cocaine is becoming a drug of commerce in the entertainment world."

Cocaine has become such a serious problem in Hollywood that film studios have started organizing against the drug. MGM/UA and the Burbank Studios recently started clinics for employees with drug or alcohol problems, Columbia is about to open its own clinic, and other studios are considering various anti-drug plans. Paramount Pictures president Michael Eisner says his studio's policy is to summon police whenever drug use is suspected; Universal's general manager Dan Slusser says a team of studio executives cooperated with the Los Angeles Police Department to investigate possible drug use on the set of a popular TV series.

Movie executives have expressed keen interest in an industry-wide program to combat drug abuse. Along with representatives from virtually every major studio, craft guild, union, and independent production company, they organized a conference early in 1984 to formulate a unified approach to misuse of cocaine and other drugs by technicians, actors, and other industry workers.

NEW HOLLYWOOD PICTURE: "COKE PLUS..."

As if cocaine were not by itself enough of a problem to California's fast-moving superstars, it is being seen more and more in combination with other popular drugs.

Marijuana and cocaine together are gaining wide acceptance at parties, with marijuana the drug of choice for most of the evening, followed by a cocaine nightcap. The coke kicker is said to combat marijuana's major side effect, tiredness, and help people drive home safely.

Most subscribers to the combination fail to realize, however, that while coke will make them more alert, it will *not* improve muscular reflexes dulled by hours of puffing marijuana. If an out-of-control auto careens toward them, they may realize instantly what is happening but lack the coordination to do anything about it.

Another stylish combination is coke and "'ludes." Methaqualone (Quaalude), a tranquilizer, "takes the edge off" a cocaine high, users say, but doesn't diminish its intensity. Some enthusiasts gulp down close to a dozen Quaalude tablets in the course of a day, to "balance" their cocaine intake.

Yet methaqualone itself is both physically and psychologically dangerously addictive and regular high doses can lead to a variety of health problems, sometimes ending in death. The two drugs in combination have not been studied extensively enough for researchers to say with certainty that there are no hidden dangers to their use.

Perhaps the most dangerous cocaine combination is the "speedball," where coke and heroin—or some other depressant—are joined together by snorting, injecting, or smoking. While the cocaine provides a high, the heroin "downer" counteracts the coke effects, seeming to make the exhilaration last longer and dampening the inevitable "lost" feeling after using cocaine.

"At least in Hollywood," said one researcher, the speedball is "a very chic thing to do." It's a "chic" combination that nearly destroyed the Phillips family of entertainers, was used by John Belushi before his death, and is implicated in the 1984 death of David Kennedy, whose body contained traces of cocaine and Demerol (synthetic heroin).

Speedballing is especially dangerous because users believe they are safe from overdose. Their hearts don't beat as fast as with coke alone, nor do they feel as agitated. Experts say the speedballer is even more likely to repeat the experience than the cocaine-alone enthusiast, but as the body builds up a tolerance to the drugs involved, overdose is more and more likely to occur.

"COKE HEADLINERS"

Today's coke *cachet* among entertainers, and in American society in general, is epitomized by the December 1983 Jodie Foster incident in Boston.

The famous 21-year-old actress, on leave from Yale University, was returning to the United States from a trip to Europe. An alert customs inspector at Boston's Logan International Airport spotted a suspicious white powder she was carrying, and asked her to identify it.

The powder was cocaine, she readily admitted. Close to a gram, in fact.

A few years ago, the discovery of cocaine—virtually any amount—in the possession of a show business personality would likely have created a media sensation. One can easily envision young prosecutors jumping at the chance to enhance their careers through the attendant publicity of arrest, indictment, and trial, and a host of defense lawyers offering their learned opinions on television talk shows, letting the world know of their availability to help rescue the actress from prison.

None of that happened.

Customs officials notified the Federal Drug Enforcement Administration of the smuggling attempt.

The federal authorities notified the United States Attorney's office.

The U.S. Attorney turned the incident over to the county district attorney.

None of the agencies wanted to prosecute the actress.

Eventually, the county D.A. released a tepid statement saying there was still a chance that charges would be filed, but it was viewed more as a face-saving gesture than a firm assertion of intent.

Jodie Foster, in the meantime, turned her cocaine over to customs agents, signed a simple document permitting the U.S. government to keep it, paid a $100 administrative fine, and walked away.

While a final outcome of Jodie Foster's run-in with drug enforcement laws is still to be determined as of this writing, the extent of her punishment appears to be the payment of a fine roughly equal to the value of the confiscated drug.

This incident is yet another signal that the use of cocaine by stars and starlets carries little more stigma than littering, running a red light, or holding a noisy party.

16
COCAINE AND SPORTS

We view athletes who excel in particular sports as nearly super-human, capable of extraordinary feats during *the* game of the year, as well as in everyday life among their family, friends, and co-workers.

When we teach our children how to hold a bat, we describe the courage and honesty of Babe Ruth, while conveniently forgetting the Babe's frequent battles with the bottle.

We argue with equal vehemence about the famous quarterback's bad pass, and his bad marriage. We squirm with the same discomfort over the loss of a home basketball game to the visiting team . . . and the death of the star player's little son in a senseless accident.

Sports figures—despite the incontrovertible fact that they are, in so many ways, much like the rest of us—have been elevated to Olympus, where only gods reside.

And we demand much of our gods. Perhaps too much. We are prone to grow vigorously angry when they let us down.

After all, we reason, they have so much more than we do: contracts worth enormous sums, an unlimited choice of friends, vast media coverage. Surely, there can be no reason for an athlete with all that to chase the added thrills of cocaine!

PUBLICITY AVALANCHE

On a statistical basis, it is unclear whether there is actually more cocaine usage in the sports world than in other professions.

Published estimates of cocaine abuse among the nation's roughly 1,500 National Football League players report that as many as 600 have experimented with the drug, a far higher percentage than among the general public. And some studies show as many as half of all pro football players use cocaine on a regular "weekend" basis, with up to ten or more "hard-core" users per team.

Ken Moffett, former executive director of the Major League Baseball Players Association, said "an awful lot" of baseball players have used cocaine. He cited reports from player representatives asserting that on some teams, as many as "four or five [players], on the average," are involved in cocaine use. Moffett also said the FBI had provided him with information about drug abuse among baseball players.

Nelson Doubleday, owner of the New York Mets, believes "the single largest problem baseball has is drugs. It is a lot more serious than people [are aware of], and it has been shoved under the rug at times."

Other research indicates the degree of drug use by sports figures is much lower than this. Regardless of the true extent of cocaine abuse in sports, whatever level does exist is clearly sufficient to bring on an avalanche of adverse publicity.

When the checkout clerk at your local supermarket is fired for using coke on the job, you'll probably never hear about it. But when a major league baseball player—who helped win the pennant two years running—is indicted on drug charges, a swarm of journalists and sports commentators quickly lays siege to the team's locker room, the owner's office, the commissioner's weekend hideaway, even the errant athlete's living room.

We are drowned with detailed reports about the star's every personal and professional move. We learn every detail of the arrest, the indictment, the trial, the sentence. And we are constantly made to wonder: Why?

PUSHED TO THE LIMIT

Often, it is the very stardom we confer on them that leads so many athletes to cocaine.

Just as we revere their playing abilities, we lavish praise on their nonsporting endeavors. Products bearing the names and faces of famous athletes outsell the competition. A fun-in-the-sun resort touting an athlete's endorsement worries little about empty rooms. Athletes sell cars, candy, and computers on television. And what they sometimes lack in acting ability, they certainly make up in easy recognition. They guest-star on television programs, and lead big-city parades.

But the majority of athletes—facing the incredible glitter of stardom—are men and women who, until their successes in sports, worried about the next mortgage payment, struggled to put their kids through school, or wondered whether they were even in the right business.

SOCIAL PRESSURE

E.J. Junior, linebacker for the St. Louis Cardinals, was convicted of cocaine possession in 1982. "Social pressures" were behind the athlete's cocaine involvement, E.J. said later. "As a pro athlete, you're always in the limelight. People are always trying to be your friends, and you don't know if they want to be your friends because you're E.J. Junior, or just because you're making lots of money."

The pressures faced by E.J. Junior ranged from a sudden spurt in income—"from the zero tax bracket the year before to the 50 percent tax bracket," he told an interviewer—as his football career flourished, to the divorce of his parents and the death of his fiancée.

Into the midst of his troubles came coke.

"Cocaine," says E.J., "gives you a good feeling."

It is easy to understand the importance of that "good feeling" for someone plagued by troubles even when, as E.J. reports, it only lasts "a very short period of time."

Also under substantial pressure was pro football lineman Carl Eller, who says cocaine "made me feel optimistic, aggressive, competent." The drug, he adds, "reinforced all of the positive things I wanted to feel about myself, things that I wasn't convinced of before."

Eller started using cocaine in the '70s as "an escape from the pressures and demands of professional football." Initially, Eller recalled years later, he was attracted to the drug partly because of "the life-style that went along with it. It was mysterious, a kind of cult, different from the mainstream. . . ."

In a few short years, cocaine use "began to catch up with me," Eller says, and it reduced his concentration and "dedication to other things. You begin to focus on the drug itself, and your other responsibilities don't get taken care of."

Cocaine "ruined my home life," he says, and "shortened my football career, perhaps by two or three years. It ruined me financially."

USA Today (August 11, 1983), editorializing on the arrest of yet another football star, Tony Peters, on charges of conspiring to sell cocaine, put the sports world's drug problem this way: "Pampered, immature athletes, intoxicated by stardom and sudden wealth, are easy prey [to the lure of cocaine].... So many [sports] stars are seduced by cocaine because it's so easy to get...[and it] creates a sense of euphoric power craved by those thrust into hero status."

BASKETBALL CASE

Football players aren't the only athletes who use cocaine to relieve pressures they are ill-prepared to face, or who find the drug easily available from those anxious to be a part of their success.

New Jersey Nets all-star guard Micheal Ray Richardson, who eventually underwent three treatment programs in just four months to kick cocaine, says he started taking the drug in response to "depression."

"I didn't know what coke would do for me," he says, "but it at least got me away from reality."

Richardson's basketball career was well under way when he was unexpectedly traded twice in a single season: from the Knicks to Golden State and then to the Nets. "I was hurt," he recalls. "I just didn't know how to deal with it."

Adding to his frustration was the departure, without advance notice to Richardson, of Nets coach Larry Brown, a close friend. Brown "just up and leaves," says the player. "That was a big letdown."

While in California, the athlete met many "so-called friends," he says, in hotels, discos—and "everywhere." They offered him free cocaine because "they just wanted to be around" the sports star. Richardson at first used coke occasionally, but was soon firmly hooked on the drug. The exhilaration of cocaine proved too strong for Richardson—as it does for so many users—and the drug's easy availability compounded the problem.

Fortunately, Richardson's story seems to be ending on a happy note. After being dropped from his team because of cocaine—and threatened with the loss of $800,000 in guaranteed salary—he was eventually reinstated under the terms of the league's new drug-abuse policies. He went on to become the star of the 1984 Nets playoff team. And when asked if he had finally kicked cocaine for good, the player said with a grin: "Yeah!"

CRYSTAL ON THE DIAMOND

Cocaine has become increasingly popular among baseball players, too. Team owners, who earlier denied there was any significant degree of coke usage among players, have been forced to become vigilant in their efforts to identify the growing legions of ballplayers involved with the drug.

In the past few years, 16 major league players have eiher been convicted of drug-related crimes, or have admitted their drug problems, and received help to control them. Another 11 players have been mentioned in drug investigations. Many other players received confidential counseling for drug abuse.

Like their counterparts in football and basketball, team executives are trying a variety of antidrug measures to slow the cocaine express. Suspension is just one weapon to keep coke users out of the game. Training sessions to teach coaches and others who deal with players on a day-to-day basis how to spot drug use among players is another.

Sometimes, cocaine not only removes a player from the game as a result of administrative action, but lands him in prison at the same time.

Willie Wilson, the Kansas City Royals star centerfielder, began a three-month jail sentence shortly before Christmas 1983, following a cocaine conviction. His sentence was generally regarded as somewhat stronger than that received by most people convicted on similar charges. A few days later, baseball commissioner Bowie Kuhn banished Wilson and three other athletes involved with drugs from the game for a full year. (An arbitrator later reinstated Wilson.)

While most professional athletes facing drug charges remain silent about the punishment dealt them by courts, and the snubs from other players, Wilson was anxious to speak out. In a series of televised interviews from his Fort Worth, Texas, penitentiary, he lashed out at the judicial system.

UNWILLING ROLE MODEL

At his sentencing, Wilson was criticized for failing to "live up to" his responsibilities as a role model and "national hero," but the athlete had other ideas. "That's a responsibility I never asked for," he complained. "All I signed a contract to do is play baseball, and that's my job."

Wilson went on: "I didn't sign a contract to take care of anybody else's kids or to be a role model for anybody else. . . . to go around taking care of millions of other kids is just something I never asked for."

Indeed, as the *New York Times* was quick to point out, the inscription above the Supreme Court Building in Washington—"Equal Justice Under Law"—says nothing "about a special brand of justice for professional baseball players." If the severity of the sentencing was due to Wilson's being a role model, said the *Times*, the judge was "presumptuous, and unfair."

Other observers of the sports scene were equally critical of the court's punishment, but somewhat more understanding of the baseball commissioner's action.

The *New York Times* stated that the commissioner "has a responsibility somewhat different" from the judge's. "Baseball markets itself as the national pastime, and [commissioner] Kuhn is representing the interests of the owners of 26 major league ball teams . . . so image is important. . . ." In the newspaper's opinion, the baseball commissioner's duty is "to protect his business."

Wilson soon had major league company in the same jail. Vida Blue, winner of the prestigious Cy Young Award and once named the American League's most valuable player, began a three-month prison term early in 1984 for cocaine possession. Blue was one of four Kansas City Royals caught in a federal cocaine investigation a few months earlier.

The "Behind-the-Bars Batters" did not include Braves pitcher Pascual Perez, who was arrested in the Dominican Republic, hundreds of miles away in the Caribbean, on a charge of possessing a small amount of cocaine with the intent to distribute it.

After pleading guilty during a preliminary hearing, Perez insisted he hadn't known the powder was coke. It was given to him by someone in Atlanta, he said, and he never realized what it was.

"I swear that I have never consumed cocaine," he proclaimed. "Neither am I a drug addict." Perez faced a possible five-year jail sentence, and a fine up to $5,000, but was convicted only of a misdemeanor in a Dominican Republic trial, and released after serving three months in prison there.

ACCEPTABLE ELIXIRS

The desire to avoid adverse cocaine publicity extends well beyond the major games of basketball, football, and baseball. Coke is equally popular in such diverse sports as horse racing, boxing, and tennis.

A Nebraska jockey—along with half a dozen track employees—was barred from racing due to his use of cocaine. Another jockey in Louisiana was suspended for possession of coke. And, in a bizarre twist to the age-old story of drugged race horses, a thoroughbred in New Orleans was shown to have coke in its bloodstream. Apparently, someone decided that the cocaine "rush" would help speed the animal to victory.

As for boxing, Aaron Pryor, the World Boxing Association's junior welterweight champion, was arrested late in 1983 for possession of cocaine. Just a few decades ago—shortly before the turn of the century—his cocaine involvement would hardly have been noteworthy. Mixtures of coke and brandy were then considered acceptable pre- and post-fight elixirs for boxers. But laws have changed, and many of today's fighters, both professional and amateur, have been accused of using or possessing cocaine. Others have been quietly disqualified from bouts by suspicious managers, trainers, or ringside physicians.

Middleweight Louis Rivera admits that, during his active career, he was high during "seven or eight of my twenty-six professional fights." Such a figure may be more common than once imagined. A New York State fight official says that "20 percent of the 360 licensed boxers are probably taking drugs at one time or another."

And Harold Weston, former welterweight contender and now "matchmaker" for Madison Square Garden, says the number could be even higher. "I wouldn't be afraid to make it about 30 percent. It seems to be getting out of hand."

The dangers of cocaine during a fight, says Dr. Edwin Campbell, medical chief of the N.Y. State Athletic Commission, stem from the drug's effects on the cardiovascular system. "Some fighters on [cocaine] can stay on a high for an entire ten-round fight," he says, "which is very hard on the heart."

In addition, coke reduces a fighter's ability to withstand punishing punches. Also, Dr. Campbell adds with classic understatement, cocaine can even "cause death sometimes."

A near scandal involving cocaine has also rocked professional tennis, a sport whose ardent fans include some of the country's most illustrious business leaders and politicians.

Individuals in touch with one major investigation, early in 1983, hinted that a number of famous players were about to be named as cocaine users, suppliers, or smugglers. While close associates of several tennis stars were eventually taken into custody, there were no arrests of notable players. Said one investigator: "We know they're using coke, we just couldn't get enough [evidence] for convictions."

Olympic sports has its own drug problems, mainly involving various chemicals that help build muscles.

But from time to time, an Olympic star's name hits the headlines in a story about cocaine.

Ken Sitzberger won a coveted Olympic gold medal in 1964 for his incredible diving. He died twenty years later under what can best be described as "suspicious circumstances." The 38-year-old athlete suffered a serious head injury—what detective novels would call a "blow to the head by an unknown object"—just weeks prior to testifying in a case against a major cocaine importing and distribution gang operating in California.

The indictment against five alleged coke kingpins says Sitzberger and an acquaintance bought cocaine themselves, and that they were also involved in burglarizing the home of a drug suspect and stealing $175,000. Details of the case have yet to emerge. The official cause of Sitzberger's death is still unknown, but it is clear that even Olympic stars are not immune to involvement with this dangerous drug.

THE AMATEUR ARENA

Just a few years ago, cocaine was rarely used by amateur sports figures. More commonly abused were such drugs as amphetamine, marijuana, and barbiturates. But just as cocaine grew popular in professional sports, it gained wide acceptance among amateurs. Over the four-year period ending in 1980, the use of coke among 18-to-25-year-olds soared by 40 percent, according to a government survey. A long-range study extending from 1962 to 1980 showed a jump in the number of youngsters who tried "hard" drugs like cocaine, from just 3 percent of the population to a full 33 percent.

According to Dr. David E. Smith, the country is in the midst of "a shift to alcohol and cocaine."

A recent Minnesota study of drug use among ninth through twelfth graders bears out the extent of stimulant abuse among student athletes. While most drugs, along with beer and wine, were used in roughly the same proportions by the entire student population, the use of stimulants like cocaine was found to be three times greater for athletes.

Amateur football, weight lifting, and track and field are spotlighted as the sports most prone to generating student drug problems. Some high schools and colleges have gone so far as to drop football from their sports programs because of continuing drug problems.

Such sports, experts say, "breed" drug abuse because of the high number of injuries they produce, injuries requiring athletes to play despite their pain, or turn to pain-relieving drugs on an ever-expanding basis. The excessive use of legitimate drugs, it is surmised, leads in some cases to the use of illicit ones.

Similar reasons exist for drug abuse among school-age athletes and their professional colleagues. Most important is peer pressure, followed by a monumental desire to be successful.

A TYPICAL CASE

Dr. Joseph A. Pursch has developed a scenario of how drug use begins among young athletes, and extends into the professional sports arena.

"Roy is the oldest child from a large family that is poor, God-fearing and strict," Dr. Pursch wrote for *USA Today*. "When he is ten, his father gives him the whipping of his life because on his way home from school, Roy cut across the mayor's lawn."

The hypothetical youngster, at twelve, becomes a Little League baseball or football sensation. "From that day on, Roy is different . . . they come in droves from surrounding towns to cheer."

But on a "psychological level something insidious begins to happen. As his value to the sport grows, his responsibility to society diminishes. We expect more and more from Roy the Star—and less and less from Roy the Man."

Breaking the mayor's window brings applause for his great throw, not reprimands. He gets away with talking back. He cuts classes. He gets drunk, and others cover up for the hero.

"Nobody levels with him anymore," Dr. Pursch writes. "He lies, and we act like it's true; he bends a rule, and we rationalize it for him; he loses his temper, and we blame others' provocations."

Roy grows up. "Emotionally immature, he is twenty—going on twelve." Headlines and big money follow. Talk-show hosts flatter him. Everybody wants to be seen with Roy.

"Happily, or so it seems, there is better living through chemistry." A pulled muscle is cured with a pill or a drink. Soon, too, is the unhappiness, with ever-stronger drugs. Once Roy is hooked—on booze, cocaine, heroin—we still ignore it. Until it's almost too late to help.

When Roy became a star, according to Dr. Pursch's scenario, "*we* became terrible role models. Except for athletic performance, we made no demands, fudged on limits and gave few guidelines. Eventually Roy became as bad a role model for us as we were for him."

USING COKE TO COPE

Carl Miller, athletic director at the University of North Dakota in Grand Forks, says college can force a young athlete to confront the fact that success may never be attained. "Suppose the star high school athlete just isn't big, fast, or strong enough to make it in college," he says.

"The day comes when the coach has to tell him. Meanwhile, of course, the kid is under enormous pressure to succeed, from his pals, from his girl friend, from everybody—nobody can face failure in our society."

The quest for financial security and educational opportunity are other factors placing stress on student athletes. "When you're talking about a $50,000 private school education," says Palo Alto, California, physician Frederick Behling, "there isn't a big difference between what a professional has at stake and what a college or high school star is looking at in terms of scholarships."

Other circumstances faced by young athletes contribute further to drug abuse.

"Athletes usually are housed together as a segregated group," says Dr. Gerald Sherman, chairman of the department of pharmacology at the University of Toledo, Ohio. The segregation, Dr. Sherman believes, adds "to the isolation from general society and in part contributes to the failure of some athletes to acquire effective coping skills. This failure frequently leads to the use of drugs . . . in an attempt to escape the existence of problem situations."

"It's hard growing up," agrees Dr. Oakley Ray, who heads the mental health and behavioral sciences unit of Veterans Administration Medical Center in Nashville.

"If drugs are around, they're an easy way to deal with problems. If you're twelve or thirteen and the choice is doing drugs and having that nice, easy time, or going through the real anxiety-ridden problems of growing up—like learning to talk to girls—I think a lot of youngsters are going to do drugs."

Summarizes Dr. Ray: "Drugs wind up preventing many things from happening that should happen in those early adolescent years."

A LIFE OF UNREALITY

Drug abuse is frequently made easier for young athletes, experts say, by so-called "enablers," friends or family members—even coaches or trainers—who for a variety of reasons keep the individual away from such realities of life as losing a game, or failing a test. These "enablers" might help convince a college football player, say, that poor grades are unimportant but winning the next game is essential.

This type of friendly, but misdirected, guidance twists the athlete's priorities so badly, say experts, that when faced with the decision to accept or refuse cocaine, they have no built-in psychological barrier to the drug's use.

Giving young athletes—or young people in general—the facts about cocaine is unlikely, in itself, to result in their avoiding the drug. "The decision to use drugs," says one researcher, "is not based on facts. It is based on life-style and on our whole orientation to the things around us."

At the end of a speech about the dangers of drugs delivered before an audience of athletes, a drug-abuse specialist was astounded when several of them approached him afterwards seeking recommendations on the best drugs to use.

A survey of Purdue University students found that knowing about the dangers of alcohol did not change the student body's use of it. Another study, this one at Vanderbilt University, showed that students pay little attention to warnings about drugs.

Adding to the problem is the continuing lack of knowledge about cocaine among high school and college sports officials. While professional teams are beginning to face the burdens imposed on them by coke, many of their counterparts in amateur athletics still insist the drug represents no significant danger to their schools, players, or team images.

"Half of the college coaches" in one survey "clung to the unrealistic belief that no member of their team used marijuana," one of the most commonly employed illegal substances in popular use today, says a report in *The Physician and Sportsmedicine*. "Few coaches at any level thought their clubs included any problem drinkers or players who had ever tried cocaine, despite persuasive statistical evidence to the contrary."

PLACED ON PEDESTALS

There exist two vastly different ways to look at cocaine use by major sports figures. We can regard baseball, football, and basketball players as mere employees who work for companies which seek profit through ticket sales to their games. The players themselves, in this view, are much like Detroit assembly-line workers. They put in a day's work and receive whatever wages are normally paid for their talents.

The individual who tightens an almost-identical bolt hundreds of times daily cannot be expected to feel any particular obligation to be a model of propriety to all those who eventually buy autos. If the laborer wants the kick of cocaine from time to time, can there be any genuine reason for the occasional use of drugs to be turned into a media sensation?

Similarly, the athlete, a worker with special skills fitted to his or her particular game, is under no obligation to show super-human character when faced with financial difficulties, family problems, or emotional turmoil. Why should the occasional use of drugs like cocaine be cause for controversy?

Since *we* are the ones who place crowns on their heads, *we* are the ones who must be satisfied with the athletes' conduct. We condone a strange twist in notions of personal freedom and individual responsibility. While assuring each other that everyone must "sleep in the bed he makes himself," we sports fans still insist on stripping every element of privacy from athletes. We expect the world of our sports stars, and loudly grieve when they fail to meet our standards.

PROFESSIONAL SPORTS AND DRUGS
Summaries of the anti-drug positions of professional sports organizations.

NATIONAL FOOTBALL LEAGUE

- Players who voluntarily seek help will not be punished. Their names will remain confidential, and their club will assume costs of drug treatment.
- Players who become involved in legal difficulties because of drug use would be subject to fines and/or suspension.
- The player's union agrees with this policy.

MAJOR LEAGUE BASEBALL

- Players who voluntarily seek help will be put on probation and may be required to undergo testing to detect drug use, to enter aftercare programs, and engage in community service.
- Players convicted of a crime related to drug distribution face suspensions for at least one year and possibly for life.
- Players helping others obtain or use drugs may be suspended for one year to life.
- Any player convicted of drug possession will be suspended for one year without pay, as will players possessing or using drugs on the playing field or anywhere within a stadium.
- Once disciplined under the drug policy, any player found to violate the policy again, may be permanently barred from pro baseball.

NATIONAL BASKETBALL ASSOCIATION

- Any player who voluntarily seeks help will receive treatment under the auspices of the Life Extension Institute. The player's club will assume the cost of treatment and the player will not be disciplined in any way, and will continue to be paid his salary.
- Any player—after previously requesting and receiving treatment for a drug problem—who again comes forward voluntarily for such treatment will be suspended without pay for the period of treatment. There will not be any additional disciplinary actions.
- Any subsequent illegal use of drugs—even if voluntarily disclosed—shall result in immediate permanent dismissal from the NBA.
- Any player who is convicted of, or pleads guilty to, a crime involving heroin or cocaine shall be immediately and permanently dismissed from the NBA.
- An independent expert experienced in detection and enforcement of drug abuse shall determine if there is a reasonable cause, based on information given to

the NBA or Player's Association, to administer tests for drug use over a six-week period. These tests are to be given at the discretion of the NBA and without prior knowledge of the player.

- The National Basketball Association and the National Basketball Player's Association collaborated in the creation of this drug program.

NATIONAL HOCKEY LEAGUE

- NHL President John A. Ziegler, Jr. states, "... If you choose to be involved with illegal drugs, you will not be involved with the NHL. To any who now use or may want to use illegal drugs, we say this: 'We do not want you, get out and stay out of our business.'"

17
COCAINE IN THE BOARD ROOM

A Wall Street securities trader continues to use cocaine at work, yet he cannot recall an $18 million trade he made while high on the drug.

His is not an isolated case.

"Doing" coke on the job is no longer the exclusive province of Hollywood and the sports arena.

In the 1980s, cocaine in the workplace is a fact of life throughout all levels of American business and industry: on the assembly line, in airline hangars, on construction sites, in nuclear-power plants, at sea on oil drilling rigs, in chemical plants, and in executive board rooms.

Cocaine use at work is already widespread, and most observers of the drug scene in the United States believe it will become even more so.

Until the end of the '70s, cocaine was the "high society" drug. Its usage, and the resultant press coverage, glamorized coke. The drug soon acquired the reputation of enhancing creativity and improving performance. It carried the mystique that "everything can be done better with coke."

Today, just as the "in" crowd begins to sour on cocaine, the drug is spreading at an explosive speed through all walks of American life, including business and industry. The democratization of coke is cited as one of the major reasons American productivity is falling behind that of other important industrialized nations. And cocaine is also blamed for billions of dollars of annual business and industry losses through sick days, poor performance, and for other reasons.

THE NEW "DOW JONES LINE"

Absenteeism, lateness, theft, an increased accident rate, and irrational decisions by workers and bosses alike also contribute to the losses. Some companies will not allow their executives to make decisions after their lunch breaks, for fear they added a cocaine "chaser" to sandwiches and a beer.

One example of the way costs spiral because of cocaine: A high-tech Silicon Valley company intentionally overproduces because managers know that much of the output will be spoiled by spaced-out workers snorting cocaine from microscope slides.

The *Wall Street Journal* tells of the problem's scope within the financial arena:

> Under the influence of the drug, brokers and traders may make rash decisions and refuse to alter them because they cannot believe they are wrong. "When a position goes against you, you may double your exposure rather than get out of the market," says Frank, a professional trader in Chicago who speculates for his own account. Good money chasing after bad recently cost another trader $8,500 in 15 minutes. "Adding to a losing trade violates the No. 1 rule of trading," this man says, "but I was real coked up."

Such diverse publications as the *National Law Journal*, the *Wall Street Journal*, and all three major newsweeklies published articles recently on the use of illicit drugs, and especially cocaine, on the job. They also documented the truth that cocaine is so widespread at work that neither industry nor business can afford to ignore it any longer.

COST TO SOCIETY

Not only does drug use on the job increase the direct and indirect costs to a company and its customers, it also hurts morale and, in the end, endangers the competitive future of American business.

The profile of today's typical cocaine user is a man or woman, from twenty to thirty-nine in age, earning upwards of $25,000 yearly. And a national survey by the polling firm of Yankelovich, Skelly and White found that blue-collar workers are today more likely than professionals to have tried cocaine.

This is not surprising, considering that monotony makes many blue-collar jobs unbearably boring. Coke, together with other drugs, is used to combat the boredom, and its accompanying stress. In some factories it is snorted as commonly as coffee breaks are taken.

Outside the factory, cocaine is also prevalent. A taxi driver shot up cocaine in his cab, until a serious accident put him and the vehicle out of commission. The Rancho Seco nuclear-power plant in California faced an extensive investigation after a quarter of a gram of cocaine was discovered on a laborer.

There are no comprehensive figures available on coke use in any specific industry, but the implications of government estimates and private studies are startling. They indicate that as large a percentage of laborers use cocaine as the percentage of coke users among the general population.

In 1982, the latest year for which nationwide statistics are available, more than 22 million Americans used cocaine out of a total 12-years-or-older population of 182.5 million. This represents roughly 12 percent of the adult and young adult population of the country. And surveys show continuing increases in the percentages.

This all spells out a grim reality: there are countless accidents and enormous tragedies just waiting to happen around the country because of cocaine. Assuming there is some truth to Murphy's Law, which states whatever *can* go wrong, *will* go wrong, consider the possibilities for disaster when an airline ground crew is high on cocaine. It's not a reassuring thought if you're about to board an airplane.

THE BIG QUESTION: WHY?

An attorney used to snort cocaine from his desk drawer through a hollowed-out ballpoint pen. Lip balms are disguised cocaine vials. Salespeople take cocaine to help them deliver more hype and sell more products. Cocaine makes them all feel better, more powerful, in control.

According to Vertell Pendleton, a Chicago drug-abuse specialist and former drug user: "With cocaine you are indestructible, perfect, the giant of your dreams." Adds another former user: "Cocaine is ego food. It feeds the ego like nothing I've ever seen in my life."

Dr. Joseph Pursch says the "particular property of cocaine is that it removes fatigue and makes the user feel very optimistic, very smart, and very clever." It provides, he adds, "a burst of energy, yet it doesn't make you slur your words or stumble. And you can get all these goodies without anyone even knowing, unless you forget to dust the cocaine off your mustache."

Those very properties for which people rely on cocaine are also the drug's psychologically addicting powers, Dr. Pursch says. A cocaine user feels he or she cannot do anything any longer without the drug's help. "Coke is the drug for over-achievers," asserts another drug expert interviewed by the *Wall Street Journal*.

The newspaper's claim that "cocaine became the drug of choice in the financial community in the middle to late 1970s" shocked, but did not surprise, the financial community. Some financial observers had long suspected that drug use was tied somehow to the ups and downs of the stock market. A decline in cocaine use accompanied the Bear Market of 1980–81, according to one market analyst, but when the Bull Market began in 1982, cocaine reappeared in a big way.

Cocaine would seem to be the perfect drug for the pace and high-rolling atmosphere of a Wall Street brokerage house, where some brokers may need reinforcement to face the mob on the chaotic trading floor.

"It makes me feel mildly indestructible," says one 28-year-old trader, who adds: "It gives me a shot of energy, sort of like a bull snorting and hoofing the ground ready to attack a matador."

Another broker confesses: "You go to war every day in this business . . . you do a line [of cocaine] and you think, it's showtime! I'm ready, fans!"

The *Wall Street Journal* reported widespread cocaine use among executives, brokers, and clerical workers entrusted with millions of dollars worth of negotiable paper in every financial district in the nation. The day-to-day pressures on a stock broker who makes perhaps $100,000 a year are similar to those felt by the auto salesman who earns less than a quarter as much. Thus cocaine is just as appealing and just as useful in coping with either job.

Many brokers, traders, lawyers, and executives who snort cocaine "are making costly mistakes in business judgment," the newspaper concludes. "Sometimes, they end up wrecking promising careers. Sometimes they end up dead."

The typical day of a corporate financial executive at one New York securities firm starts with an early-morning "toot" to get going, frequent use during the day to keep up the energy, and social use in the evening, usually while entertaining clients. A former financial-community coke user says: "Every trading desk on Wall Street is full of cocaine."

In other businesses, cocaine use is similar. In one major East Coast city, an electronics-equipment manufacturer found his sales force was no longer taking customers out for drinks. Instead, they were furnishing them with coke.

A bond trader talks of "occasionally" receiving a gram or two of cocaine from people wishing to keep his "friendship." The gifts seem to work. Overly favorable ratings are sometimes given "in return for a cocaine kickback," says *Newsweek* magazine.

Another type of kickback was offered at a carpet store, whose owners provided cocaine to employees for working eighteen-hour shifts.

Cocaine use in the workplace often leads to theft from the workplace. Authorities believe that most thefts in California's computer-manufacturing region are cocaine related. Not only is the expensive coke habit the reason for theft, but the drug is also frequently the means of payment for stolen goods. "A ton of cocaine a year is consumed" in Silicon Valley, according to observers, a quantity requiring a lot of theft, by a lot of workers.

18
COCAINE AND THE LAW

In 1970, the federal government enacted The Controlled Substance Act (Public Law–91-513), which was intended to halt the spread of drugs with abuse potential and create some consistency among the more than fifty different federal types of drug regulation. Cocaine, marijuana, heroin, LSD, PCP, and all prescription pills and drugs are regulated by this act, its amendments, and other state regulations.

The main sections of the federal law establish five categories, or "schedules," which classify a drug according to its potential danger and set fines and prison terms accordingly. The law establishes separate penalties for *trafficking* and *possession*. Penalties for Schedule I violations are the harshest (Schedule I includes heroin, marijuana, LSD). Schedule V drugs are the least dangerous and are mixtures of narcotic and non-narcotic ingredients, e.g., the antidiarrheal drug Lomotil. (See Appendix A for more information).

Trafficking, in general, is a felony and is defined as the unauthorized manufacture or possession of a controlled substance with intent to sell. A felony is usually a crime punishable by at least one year in jail and/or a large fine.

Possession in most cases, but not in all, is considered to be a misdemeanor, and generally punishable by imprisonment for less than a year, and/or a fine. Often the difference between a possession and a trafficking charge is determined by the amount of the drug the suspect possessed at the time of arrest and the number of previous offenses. Further complicating the drug laws are plea bargains, or additional charges, including weapons possession, which may accompany the drug charge.

Cocaine is controlled by both federal and state laws. Federally, and medically, cocaine is classified as a Schedule II drug. This means that while it does have legitimate medical uses, it also has great potential for abuse. Drugs also included in Schedule II are barbiturates and amphetamine.

Possession of Schedule II drugs is allowed only under rigid guidelines which severely restrict prescription use. Despite the restrictions on Schedule II drugs (for example, they can't be prescribed over the phone), many are widely abused. One good example is methaqualone (Quaalude) which was widely abused, later banned by many states, and is no longer manufactured in the U.S. In cases like this, despite the medical indications of the drug, the government will reclassify such a drug to Schedule I when wide abuse is reported.

Unfortunately, there are a large number of inconsistencies between the state and federal regulations. There are no uniform state drug laws, either. States are free to set any penalties they wish and often they are much harsher than federal laws.

State laws restricting cocaine and the penalties set by these laws vary considerably. They change so rapidly that the only sure way to know each state's penalties is to check with the Office of the State Attorney General.

The bottom line is that cocaine possession by anyone other than a doctor or pharmacist is illegal. It is also illegal to use it any time, except under medical supervision.

BOOK LAW vs. COMMON PRACTICE

The reality of drug law enforcement, as individuals' personal experience and the media have shown, is that many people use coke, are arrested, but *don't* go to jail. This is in part because the circumstances under which people are found with the drug vary widely and so do community attitudes.

Often, so-called "community standards" will determine how severely a drug arrest and/or a conviction is viewed by the courts. A good example is the variation of marijuana possession laws. In some places, like New York City, pot possession is often considered as light an offense as a parking ticket. But in other areas one can go to jail for years for marijuana possession. The same attitude applies to cocaine.

Community standards are applied in circumstances where drug use is evident, but the "nature of the crime" is somewhat unclear. For example, if someone overdoses on cocaine and is taken to an emergency room, who will be notified? What will happen to the person?

First, his or her parents or next of kin may be notified if treatment is required and the patient is unable to give authorization. Hospitals generally are required to notify the police if the drug overdose was a result of a suicide attempt. Usually, police are informed of narcotic possessions, but unless they have reason to suspect the victim is a dealer or in possession of large amounts of the drug, the victim is not prosecuted.

In these cases, police and even the medical staff may apply community standards, that is, how the people in the town or city feel about the drug taken, before they decide to investigate further.

Many times a "celebrity" victim may be treated differently—either harsher or easier—depending on the attitude of local authorities. Some experts believe that athletes and other celebrities are now being prosecuted *more* than "civilians," to set an example.

But, what happens if someone is walking down the street with friends who are stopped by a policeman (for probable cause) and they are found with cocaine?

While it is not a crime to be with someone who has an illegal drug, the policeman may legally arrest all persons present. This is common practice and police tend to decide who to charge *after* they arrest people in these situations. Prosecution can follow if the bystander was present when the coke was bought—again, depending on local laws and practices.

The concept of possession and conspiracy to possess is very controversial. For example, someone may be charged if he or she discusses illegal possession of drugs but doesn't participate. It's best to avoid even participating in "what-if" sessions about drug dealing or possession. Again, community attitudes often are applied by authorities in these cases.

The individual does have rights, of course. For example, a policeman cannot search someone who is simply walking down the street. There can be no search unless there's something that arouses the policeman's suspicion or if he's actually made an arrest. If a driver is stopped while in his car, and unless drugs are in plain sight or it is a suspicious vehicle, no search may take place. (However, recent rulings by the U.S. Supreme Court may change the way police deal with auto searches and the questioning of auto passengers and drivers.)

But again, remember that cocaine is an illegal substance and the choice to possess it anywhere outside medical supervision may result in arrest and imprisonment.

The following are a few examples of how widely state laws vary for coke use or dealing.

Alaska—Possession of any amount: 1st offense, 5 years maximum and a fine; 2nd offense, 2–5 years and a fine; 3rd offense, 3–5 years and a fine. Sale of any amount: 1st offense, maximum 10 years and a fine; 2nd offense, 4–10 years and a fine; 3rd offense, 6–10 years and a fine. Delivery to anyone under 19 years of age may result in a sentence of 5–99 years and a fine of up to $75,000.

California—Possession: 1st offense, may qualify (several conditions must be met) for probation of 6 months–2 years maximum; 2nd offense, 16 months, 2 years or 3 years. Possession for sale of any amount regardless of offenses, 2, 3 or 4 years. Sale of any amount regardless of offenses, 3, 4 or 5 years.

Florida—Possession: 1st offense, 5 years maximum and a fine; 2nd offense, 10 years maximum. Sale: 1st offense, 15 years maximum and a fine; 2nd offense, 30 years maximum.

Illinois—Number of offenses not considered. Possession of under 30 grams, 1–3 years; over 30 grams, 4–15 years. Sale of up to 10 grams, 3–7 years and a fine; 10–30 grams, 4–15 years and a fine; over 30 grams, 6–30 years and a fine.

Massachusetts—Possession: 1st offense, maximum 10 years and a fine; 2nd offense, 3–10 years and a fine. Sale: 1st offense, 1–10 years and a fine; 2nd offense, 3–10 years and a fine.

New York—Possession of up to ⅛ ounce, maximum 1 year; above ⅛ ounce, 1 year to life, depending on amount. Sale: depending on amount, 1 year to life. Fines: $5,000 or double the money illicitly earned.

Texas—Possession: 1st offense, 2–20 years and a fine; 2nd offense, 5–99 years and a fine. Sale: 1st offense, 5–99 years and a fine; 2nd offense, 15–99 years.

APPENDIX A

Abbreviated Schedule of Controlled Substances: Federal Classification*

Schedule I	Schedule II	Schedule III	Schedule IV	Schedule V
NARCOTIC ANALGESICS Acetylmethadol (LAAM) Heroin STIMULANTS Amphetamine variants HALLUCINOGENS Analogs of phencyclidine Ibogaine Lysergic acid-25 (LSD) Marijuana, Hashish Mescaline Peyote Psilocybin, Psilocyn Tetrahydro-cannabinols	NARCOTIC ANALGESICS Alphaprodine Anileridine Codeine Dihydrocodeine Ethylmorphine Etorphine (M99) Fentanyl Hydrocodone Hydromorphone Levorphanol Meperidine (Pethidine) Methadone Morphine Opium Oxycodone Oxymorphone Phenazocine DEPRESSANTS Amobarbital Methaqualone Secobarbital Pentobarbital STIMULANTS Amphetamine Cocaine Methamphetamine Methylphenidate Phenmetrazine HALLUCINOGENS Phencyclidine	NARCOTIC ANALGESICS Acetaminophen + codeine APC + codeine Aspirin + codeine Nalorphine Paregoric DEPRESSANTS Any compound containing an unscheduled drug and: Amobarbital Secobarbital Pentobarbital Glutethimide Methyprylon STIMULANTS Benzphetamine Clortermine Mazindol Phendimetrazine	DEPRESSANTS Barbital Chloral betaine Chloral hydrate Chlordiazepoxide Clonazepam Clorazepate Diazepam Ethchlorvynol Ethinamate Fenfluramine Flurazepam Meprobamate Mephobarbital Oxazepam Paraldehyde Pentazocine Phenobarbital Propoxyphene Prazepam STIMULANTS Diethylpropion Phentermine Pemoline	Mixtures containing limited quantities of narcotic drugs, with non-narcotic active medicinal ingredients. Less abuse potential than Schedule IV. Generally for antitussive and antidiarrheal purposes. May be distributed without a prescription order.

*This table is based on federal regulations. State regulations may result in different classifications.

APPENDIX B

COCAINE SLANG

- Bernice
- Blow
- C
- Candy
- Carrie
- Champagne of drugs
- Coke
- Crystal
- Flake
- Free-base
- Freeze
- Gift of the Sun God
- Gold dust
- Happy dust
- Hayo (old Caribbean name for coca plant)
- Icing
- La Dama Blanca
- Lady
- Leaf
- Mama Coca (Incan name for coca plant)
- Pasta
- Pearl
- Pimp's drug
- Rich man's drug
- She
- Snow
- Stardust
- Vitamin "C"
- White Lady

APPENDIX C

COCAINE TREATMENT CENTERS

(Listed by State)

(Please note the following information is subject to change.)

NATIONAL HOTLINE
800-COCAINE
Fair Oaks Hospital
Summit, New Jersey
1-800-COCAINE

ALABAMA

Claudio Toro, M.D.,
Medical Director
Hillcrest Hospital
6869 Fifth Avenue, South
Birmingham, Alabama
35212
205-833-9000

John Cranton, M.D.,
Medical Director
(Charter) Southland Hospital
P.O. Box 7897
Mobile, Alabama 36607
205-432-8811

Edward G. Feller, M.D.
University of Southern
Alabama Medical Center
2451 Fillingin Street
Mobile, Alabama 36617
205-471-7477

ALASKA

Frank Moran, M.D.
Medical Director
Charter North Hospital
2530 DeBarr Road
Anchorage, Alaska 99508
907-338-7575

ARIZONA

Robert Mayer, M.D.
Phoenix Camelback Hospital
5055 North 34th Street
Phoenix, Arizona 85018
602-941-7509

Dennis C. Westin, M.D.,
Medical Director
Palo Verde Hospital
801 South Prudence Road
Tucson, Arizona 85710
602-298-3363

ARKANSAS

Donald Butts, M.D.,
Medical Director
Charter Vista Hospital
P.O. Box 1906
Fayetteville, Arkansas 72702
501-521-5731

Karen Keller,
Program Director
RESTORE
Riverview Medical Center
1310 Cantrell Road
Little Rock, Arkansas 72201
501-376-1200

CALIFORNIA

David B. Bergman, M.D.,
Medical Director
Southwood Mental Health Center
950 Third Avenue
Chula Vista, California 92011
619-426-6310

Ms. Ann Munoz,
Director, Renewal Unit
Dominguez Valley Hospital
3100 Susana Road
Compton, California 90221
213-639-2664

John P. Feighner, M.D.,
Medical Director
San Luis Rey Hospital
1015 Devonshire Drive
Encinitas, California 92024
619-753-1234

Richard Rawson, Ph.D.,
Director
Cocaine Associates
9033 Wilshire Boulevard
Suite 203
Beverly Hills, California 90211
213-275-9994

Namir F. Damlouji, M.D.,
Murray H. Rosenthal, D.O.
Psychiatric Centers at San Diego
P.O. Box 1660
La Mesa, California 92041
619-464-1982

Mr. David Leblanc
Doctor's Hospital of Lakewood
Clark Avenue Division
5300 N. Clark Avenue
Lakewood, California 90712
213-866-9711

Sidney Cohen, M.D.
13020 Sky Valley Road
Los Angeles, California 92041
213-472-9412

Dixon Young, M.D.,
Director, Renewal Unit, 3rd Floor
Century City Hospital
2070 Century Park East
Los Angeles, California 90067
213-277-4248

Ms. Mary McNally,
Director, Renewal Unit
Renewal Hospital of Ojai
1306 A Maricopa Highway
Ojai, California 93023
805-646-5567

Ms. Vel Gilbert,
Director, Renewal Unit
Ontario Community Hospital
550 N. Monterey
Ontario, California 91764
714-984-2201

Ms. C.J. Hawkins,
Director, Renewal Unit
Doctor's Hospital of Pinole
2151 Appian Way
Pinole, California 94564
415-724-5000

Ms. Pat Gallagher,
Director, Renewal Unit
Alisal Community Hospital
333 N. Sanborn Road, Box 2159
Salinas, California 93902
408-424-0381

Alan Adler, M.D.,
Medical Director
Alvarado Parkway Institute
5555 Reservoir Drive, Suite 206
San Diego, California 92120
619-583-2111

Robert A. Moore, M.D.,
Clinical Director
Vista Hill Foundation
3420 Camine del Rio North
San Diego, California
619-563-1770

David Smith, M.D.,
Director
Haight-Ashbury Free Clinic
409 Clayton Street
San Francisco, California 94117
415-626-6763

Brian Gould, M.D.
Walnut Creek Hospital
175 La Casa Via
Walnut Creek, California 94598
415-933-7990

COLORADO

Robert P. Snead, M.D.,
Medical Director
Boulder Psychiatric Institute
3000 Pearl Street
Boulder, Colorado 80301
303-441-0526

Richard Bangert,
Administrator
Cedar Springs Psychiatric Hospital
2135 Southgate Road
Colorado Springs, Colorado 80906
303-633-4114

Thomas Crowley, M.D.,
Professor of Psychiatry
University of Colorado School of Medicine
1827 Gaylord
Denver, Colorado 80206
303-388-5894

William W. McCaw, M.D.,
Medical Director
Mount Airy Psychiatric Center
4455 East 12th Avenue
Denver, Colorado 80220
303-322-1803

CONNECTICUT

Roger Meyer, M.D.
University of Connecticut
School of Medicine
University of Connecticut
Health Center
Farmington, Connecticut
06032
203-674-3423

Michael Sheehy, M.D.,
Medical and Executive
Director
Silver Hill Foundation, Inc.
P.O. Box 1177, 208 Valley
Rd.
New Canaan, Connecticut
06840
203-966-3561

Charles Riordan, M.D.,
Director, Substance Abuse
Unit
Connecticut Mental Health
Center
34 Park Avenue
New Haven, Connecticut
06510
203-789-7282

Lane Ameen, M.D.,
Medical Director
Elmcrest Psychiatric Institute
25 Marlborough Street
Portland, Connecticut 06480
203-342-0480

DELAWARE

Cor DeHart, M.D.,
Medical Director
Rockford Center
1605 North Broom Street
Wilmington, Delaware
19806
302-652-3892

WASHINGTON, D.C.

Marc Hertzman, M.D.
Department of Psychiatry
George Washington
University
Burns Building, 10th Floor
2150 Pennsylvania Ave.,
N.W.
Washington, D.C. 20037
202-676-3355

Howard Hoffman, M.D.,
Medical Director
Psychiatric Institute of
Washington
4460 MacArthur Boulevard,
N.W.
Washington, D.C. 20037
202-467-4600

FLORIDA

Psychiatric Institute of
Delray
5440 Linton Boulevard
Delray Beach, Florida 33445
305-495-1000

Dr. Christopher Mahon
Coral Ridge Psychiatric
Hospital
4545 North Federal Highway
Fort Lauderdale, Florida
33308
305-777-2711

Theodore J. Machler, M.D.,
Medical Director
Medfield Center
12891 Seminole Boulevard
Largo, Florida 33544
813-581-8757

Dominic Zucchro, Ph.D.,
Program Director
Lake Hospital of the Palm
Beaches
1710 Fourth Avenue North
Lake Worth, Florida 33460
305-588-7341

Roberto Cuesta, M.D.
P.L. Dodge Memorial
Hospital
2298 S.W. Eighth Street
Miami, Florida 33135
305-643-2511

Stephen Kahn, M.D.,
Medical Director of the
Recovery Center
Highland Park General
Hospital
1660 Northwest 7th Court
Miami, Florida 33136
305-326-7008

Steve Targum, M.D.
Sarasota Palms Hospital
1650 South Osprey Avenue
Sarasota, Florida 33579
813-366-6070

GEORGIA

Ronald Bloodworth, M.D.
Psychiatric Institute of
Atlanta
811 Juniper Street, N.E.
Atlanta, Georgia 30308
404-881-5800

Mr. Al Stines, Director
Substance Abuse Unit
Charter Lake Hospital
P.O. Box 7067
Macon, Georgia 31209
912-474-6200

Charter By The Sea
2927 Demese Rd
St. Simon's Island, Georgia
31522
912-638-1999

Conway Hunter, M.D.
Box 802
Cottage 328
Sea Island, Georgia 31561
912-638-2141

Mark Gould, M.D.,
Medical Director
Brawner Psychiatric Institute
3180 Atlanta Street, S.E.
Smyrna, Georgia 30080
404-436-0081

HAWAII

Lenore Sheldon,
Director
Drug Addiction Services of
Hawaii
640 Kakoi Street
Honolulu, Hawaii 96819
808-836-2330

IDAHO

Ms. Gail Ater,
Director
The Walker Center
P.O. Box 541
Gooding, Idaho 83330
208-934-8461

Mr. Eugene Cwalinski,
Director
Substance Abuse Unit
Mercy Medical Center Care
Unit
1512 12th Avenue Road
Nampa, Idaho 83651
208-466-4531

ILLINOIS

Sidney Schnoll, M.D.,
Director
Chemical Dependency Unit
Northwestern Memorial
Hospital
320 East Huron
Chicago, Illinois 60611
312-649-8713

Charlie Schuster, M.D.
University of Chicago
Department of Psychiatry
5841 South Maryland
Chicago, Illinois 60637
312-962-6360

Leo I. Jacobs, M.D.,
Medical Director
Rudolph G. Novick, M.D.,
Psychiatrist-In-Chief
Forest Hospital
555 Wilson Lane
Des Plaines, Illinois 60016
312-635-4100

INDIANA

Alden Hvidston, Director
Chemical Dependency Unit
St. Vincent's Stress Center
8401 Harcourt Road
Indianapolis, Indiana 46260
317-875-4710

IOWA

Barbara Martens, Business
Coordinator
Sedlacek Treatment Center
c/o Mercy Hospital
701 Tenth Street, S.E.
Cedar Rapids, Iowa 52403
319-398-6226

KANSAS

Robert Conroy, M.D.
C.F. Menninger Memorial
Hospital
3616 West Seventh Street
P.O. Box 829
Topeka, Kansas 66601
913-273-7500

KENTUCKY

Dr. Van Nostrand,
President, Medical Staff
Our Lady of Peace Hospital
202 Newburg Road
Louisville, Kentucky 40232
502-451-3330

LOUISIANA

Rudolph Ehrensing, M.D.
Ochsner Clinic
1514 Jefferson Highway
New Orleans, Louisiana
70121
504-838-4025

Robert Lancaster, M.D.,
Medical Director
Depaul Hospital
1040 Calhoun St.
New Orleans, Louisiana
70118
504-899-8282

Stanley Roskind, M.D.,
Medical Director
Jo Ellen Smith Psychiatric
Hospital
4601 Patterson Road
New Orleans, Louisiana
70114
504-363-7676

Gene Usdin, M.D.,
Professor of Psychiatry
Louisiana State University
1403 Delachaise Street
New Orleans, Louisiana
70115
504-891-7000

MAINE

Stanley J. Evans, M.D.,
P.A., Medical Director
Mercy Hospital Alch.
Institute
Portland, Maine 04101
207-774-1566

MARYLAND

John P. Docherty, M.D.
7401 Westlake Terrace
Bethesda, Maryland 20817
301-469-8529

Brian Schulman, M.D.
4400 East West Highway
Suite 6
Bethesda, Maryland 20814
301-654-4221

Bruce Taylor, M.D.,
Director of Admissions
Taylor Manor Hospital
College Avenue
Ellicott City, Maryland
21043
301-465-3322

John E. Meeks, M.D.,
Medical Director
Psychiatric Institute of
Montgomery County
14901 Broschart Road
Rockville, Maryland 20850
301-251-4500

MASSACHUSETTS

Steve Mirin, M.D.,
Director Drug Dependence
Treatment
McLean Hospital
115 Mill Street
Belmont, Massachusetts
02178
617-855-2151

Dr. Bernard Gray, Executive
Director
Norman Zinberg, M.D.
Comprehensive Mental
Health Services
1643 Beacon Street
Waban, Massachusetts
02168
617-969-8870

MICHIGAN

Raymond E. Buck, M.D.,
Medical Director
Psychiatric Center of
Michigan
35031-23 Mile Road
New Baltimore, Michigan
48047
313-725-5777

Mr. Robert Kercorian,
Director, Substance Abuse
Harold E. Fox Center
900 Woodward
Pontiac, Michigan 48053
313-858-3177

Mr. Steven Hnat
Substance Abuse Unit
Henry Ford Hospital
6773 West Maple Road
West Bloomfield, Michigan
48033
313-661-6100

MINNESOTA

Daniel Anderson, Ph.D., President/Director
Hazelden
15425 Pleasant Valley Road
Center City, Minnesota 55012
612-257-4010

Joseph Westermeyer, M.D.
University of Minnesota Hospital
Box 393 Mayo
420 Delaware Street, S.E.,
Minneapolis, Minnesota 55455
612-373-7952

MISSISSIPPI

Mr. Gordon McCandlish, Program Coordinator
Delta Medical Center
P.O. Box 5247
Greenville, Mississippi 38704 Box 244
601-334-2200

Mr. John Reedy, Administrator
Riverside Hospital
P.O. Box 4297
Jackson, Mississippi 39216
1-800-962-2180

MISSOURI

T.H. Boldt, M.D.
George Hamlin, Prevention/Intervention Supervisor
The Edgewood Program
St. John's Mercy Medical Center
615 S. New Ballas Rd.
St. Louis, Missouri 63141
314-569-6500

Washington University School of Medicine
Outpatient Service
4950 Audubon
St. Louis, Missouri 63110
314-362-7005

William Clary, M.D., Medical Director
Ozark Psychiatric Clinic
1900 South National, Suite 1800
Springfield, Missouri 65804
417-881-3124

MONTANA

Mr. Robert Barren, Director of Alcohol & Drug Program
St. James Hospital East
25 Continental Drive
Butte, Montana 59701
406-723-4341

Mr. David Cunningham, Executive Director
Rim Rock Foundation
P.O. Box 30374
Billings, Montana 59107
406-248-3175

NEBRASKA

Mr. Jim Mays, Director of Alcohol Treatment Center
Immanuel Medical Center
6901 North 72nd
Omaha, Nebraska 68122
402-572-2016

NEVADA

William Thornton, M.D.,
Medical Director
Truckee Meadows Hospital
1240 East Ninth Street
Reno, Nevada 89512
702-323-0478

Mr. Mark Augenstien
Care Unit Hospital
1401 Lake Meade Avenue
North Las Vegas, Nevada
89030
702-642-6905

NEW HAMPSHIRE

Allan Carney,
Director of RADD
Hampstead Hospital
East Road
Hampstead, New Hampshire
03841
603-329-5311

George Griffin, M.D.,
Medical Director
Spofford Hall
Box 157
Spofford, New Hampshire
03462
Out of State: 800-451-1716
In State: 603-363-4545

NEW JERSEY

Peter Mueller, M.D.
Princeton Hospital
905 Herrintown Road
Princeton, New Jersey
08540
609-924-4061

Russell Ferstandig, M.D.,
P.A.
179 S. Maple Avenue
Ridgewood, New Jersey
07450
201-445-9777

Mark Gold, M.D.,
Director of Research
Fair Oaks Hospital
1 Prospect Street
Summit, New Jersey 07901
1-800-COCAINE

Jane Jones, M.D.
Psychiatric Associates of
New Jersey
19 Prospect Street
Summit, New Jersey 07901
201-522-7000

William Vilensky, M.D.
Suite 106, Kennedy
Professional Mall
40 Laurel Road
Stratford, New Jersey 08084
609-346-7025

NEW MEXICO

John McCormack, M.D.
Vista Sandia Hospital
501 Richfield Avenue, N.E.
Albuquerque, New Mexico
87113
505-898-1661

Joel Hochman, M.D.
St. Vincent's Hospital
664 Camino Del Monte Sol
Santa Fe, New Mexico
87501
505-982-2529

NEW YORK

Robert Bertoni
Bry Lin Hospital
1263 Delaware Avenue
Buffalo, New York 14209
716-886-8200

David Steinberg, M.D.
Falkirk Psychiatric Hospital
P.O. Box 194
Central Valley, New York 10917
914-928-2256

Joel Solomon, M.D.
300 West End Avenue,
New York, New York 10023
212-595-9119

Arnold Washton, Ph.D.
Metropolitan Medical Group
425 East 61st Street
New York, New York 10021
212-935-3400

Stuart Yudovsky, M.D.
Stony Lodge Hospital
Ossining/Croton-on-Hudson
Westchester, N.Y. 10562
914-941-7400

NORTH CAROLINA

Jack W. Bonner III, M.D., Medical Director
Highland Hospital
49 Zillicoa Street, P.O. Box 1101
Asheville, North Carolina 28802
704-254-3201

Dennis Christianson, M.D., Medical Director
Appalachian Hall
P.O. Box 5534 Caledonia Road
Asheville, North Carolina 28813
704-253-3681

Everett Ellinwood, Jr., M.D.
Duke University Medical Center
Box 3870
Durham, North Carolina 27710
919-684-5225

NORTH DAKOTA

Will Wells, M.D., Clinical Director
Hartview Foundation
1406 N.W. 2nd Street
Mandan, North Dakota 58554
701-663-2321

OHIO

Bill Moore
Emerson A. North Hospital
5642 Hamilton Avenue
Cincinnati, Ohio 45224
513-541-0135

William Webber, M.D.
Woodruff Hospital
1950 East 89th Street
Cleveland, Ohio 44106
216-795-3700

OKLAHOMA

Mr. Bill Steele,
 Director, Chemical
 Dependency Unit
Presbyterian Hospital
707 N.W. 6th Street
Oklahoma City, Oklahoma
 73102
405-232-0777

Michael Dubriwny, M.D.,
 Medical Director
Shadow Mountain Institute
6262 S. Sheridan Road
Tulsa, Oklahoma 74133
918-492-8200

OREGON

Daniel Bloch, M.D.,
 Medical Director
Cedar Hills Psychiatric
 Hospital
10300 S.W. Eastridge Street
Portland, Oregon 97225
503-292-9101

PENNSYLVANIA

Ken Sandler, M.D.
The Fairmount Institute
561 Fairthorne Street
Philadelphia, Pennsylvania
 19128
215-487-4102

Jerry A. Romoff,
 Administrator
Western Psychiatric Institute
 and Clinic
3811 O'Hara Street
Pittsburgh, Pennsylvania
 15261
412-624-2000

Lyon Williams,
 Clinical Director
Marworth Hospital
Waverly, Pennsylvania
 18471
717-563-1112

RHODE ISLAND

Andrew Slaby, M.D.,
 Ph.D., Psychiatrist in
 Chief
Brown University Division
 of Biology & Medicine
Rhode Island Hospital
593 Eddy Street
Providence, Rhode Island
 02902
401-277-5488

Ming T. Tsuang, M.D.,
 Assistant Medical Director,
 Director of Research
Butler Hospital
345 Blackstone Blvd.
Providence, Rhode Island
 02906
401-456-3855

SOUTH CAROLINA

Douglas F. Crane, M.D.,
 Medical Director
Fenwick Hall
P.O. Box 688
 Maybank Highway and
 River Road
Johns Island, South Carolina
 29455
803-559-2461

Christopher Caston, M.D.
711 N. Church, Suite 110
Spartanburg, South Carolina
 29303
803-585-0328

SOUTH DAKOTA

Mr. Charles Brewer
Coordinator of Patient Care
River Park, Inc.
P.O. Box 1216
Pierre, South Dakota 57501
605-224-6177

TENNESSEE

Robert Booher, M.D.,
Medical Director
Peninsula Psychiatric
Hospital
Route #2, Box 233
Louisville, Tennessee 37777
615-573-7913

Joel Reismann, M.D.
Addictive Disease Unit
Lakeside Hospital
2911 Brunswick Rd.
Memphis, Tennessee 38134
901-377-4700

Susan Reimer, Administrator
Park View Hospital
Parthenon Pavilion
2401 Murphy Avenue
Nashville, Tennessee 37203
615-327-2237

TEXAS

Lawrence Arnold, M.D.,
Medical Director
Brookhaven Psychiatric
Pavilion
Seven Medical Parkway
Dallas, Texas 75234
214-247-1000

Mark Unterberg, M.D.,
Director of Substance
Abuse Group Program
Timberlawn Psychiatric
Hospital, Inc.
4600 Samuels Blvd.
P.O. Box 11288
Dallas, Texas 75223
214-381-7181

Frederick Goggans, M.D.
Psychiatric Associates of
Texas, Fort Worth
815 Eighth Avenue
Fort Worth, Texas 76104
817-335-4040

Lawrence Schweitzer, M.D.,
Associate Professor,
Deputy Chief of Psychiatry
Baylor College of Medicine
1200 Moorsund Avenue
Houston, Texas 77030
713-799-4892

UTAH

Donnis Reece, Ph.D.,
Program Administrator
St. Benedict's ACT Center
1255 East 3900 South
Salt Lake City, Utah 84117
801-263-1300

VERMONT

Robert Landeen, M.D.
Brattleboro Retreat
75 Linden Street
Brattleboro, Vermont 05301
800-451-4203

Mr. Norman Reuss
Champlain Drug Services
45 Clark Street
Burlington, Vermont 05401
802-863-3456

VIRGINIA

Willis G. Goodenow, M.D.
Unit Director for Chemical Dependency Treatment Program
David C. Wilson Hospital
2101 Arlington Ave.
Charlottesville, Virginia 22903
804-977-1120

Stuart Ahman, M.D., Director, Substance Abuse Unit
Serenity Lodge
2097 South Military Highway
Chesapeake, Virginia 23320
804-543-6888

C. Gibson Dunn, M.D., Medical Director
Springwood Psychiatric Institute
Route 4, Box 50
Leesburg, Virginia 22075
703-777-0800

Joseph Garten, M.D.
Psychiatric Institute of Richmond, Inc.
3001 Fifth Avenue
Richmond, Virginia 23222
804-329-4392

WASHINGTON

Elliott Oppenheim, M.D.
8430 Main Street
Edmonds, Washington 98020
206-774-5113

Kay E. Seim, Administrator
Kirkland Care Unit Hospital
10200 N.E. 132nd Street
Kirkland, Washington 98033
206-821-1122

WEST VIRGINIA

Edwin L. Johnson, Administrator
Highland Hospital
300 56th Street
Charleston, West Virginia 25304
304-925-4756

WISCONSIN

Jerry Reichert, Administrator
St. Croixdale Hospital
445 Court Street North
Prescott, Wisconsin 54021
715-262-3286

Craig Larsen, M.D., Medical Director
Milwaukee Psychiatric Hospital
Dewey Center
1220 Dewey Avenue
Wauwatosa, Wisconsin 53213
414-258-4094

WYOMING

Durward Burnett, M.D.
Substance Abuse Unit
Wyoming State Hospital
P.O. Box 177
Evanston, Wyoming 82930
307-789-3464

SOURCES

"Aides Still Sniffing Into Jodie's Coke." (N.Y.) *Daily News,* 21 December 1983.

Altman, Lawrence K. "The Private Agony Of An Addicted Physician." *New York Times,* 7 June 1983.

Anderson, Kurt. "Crashing on Cocaine." *Time,* 11 April 1983.

Anker, Antoinette L., and J. Crowley, Thomas. "Use of Contingency Contracts in Specialty Clinics for Cocaine Abuse." *NIDA Research Monograph Series 41, Problems of Drug Dependence 1981.* Proceedings of the 43rd Annual Scientific Meeting. The Committee on Problems of Drug Dependence, Inc.

Barenfeld, Steve. "Nets Reinstate Sugar: NBA Pushes Move To Prevent Problems With Drug Program." *New York Post,* 22 December 1983.

Barre, Felix. "Cocaine As An Abortive Agent In Cluster Headache." *Headache,* Vol. 22, no. 69–73 (March 1982).

Beck, Melinda, and Buckley, Jerry. "Nurses With Bad Habits." *Newsweek,* 22 August 1983.

Berkow, Ira. "Willie Wilson, Citizen." *New York Times,* 22 December 1983.

"Blue Beginning 3-Month Term." *New York Times,* 3 January 1984.

"Blue Gets 3 Months On Cocaine Charge." *New York Times,* 20 December 1983.

Brady, James. "Drugs: When The Glamor Stops." *New York Post,* 29 November 1983.

"Braves' Perez Busted For Coke." *New York Post,* 11 January 1984.

"Braves' Pitcher Held For Drugs." *New York Times,* 11 January 1984.

Brody, Jane E. "How Drugs Can Cause Decreased Sexuality." *New York Times,* 28 September 1983.

"A Brutal 'Cocaine Coup.'" *Newsweek,* 11 August 1980.

Chilnick, L.D., ed. *The Little Black Pill Book.* New York: Bantam Books, 1983.

"Cocaine Casualty." *People Weekly,* 29 August 1983.

"Cocaine Treatment Is Said To Cause Paranoia." *New York Times,* 28 October 1982.

Cohen, Sidney. "A Cocaine Primer." In *Cocaine: A Second Look*. The American Council on Marijuana and Other Psychoactive Drugs, Inc., 1983.
"Coke And No Smile." *Time*, 9 August 1982.
Colacello, Bob. "Why Jodie Foster Won't Quit." *Parade Magazine*, 11 December 1983.
Coleman, D.L., et al. "Angina and Myocardial Infarction After Recreational [Snorting] of Cocaine." *Western Journal of Medicine*, Vol. 136, no. 5 (May 1982).
"Columbia–Venezuela Accord Aimed at Drugs and Rebels." *New York Times*, 20 February 1984.
Copetas, A. Craig. "Coca Fields of Bolivia." (N.Y.) *High Times*, date unknown.
"Crashing on Cocaine." *Time*, 11 April 1983.
"DeLorean's Judge Bids Agencies Present Data." *New York Times*, 12 January 1984.
"Dependence On Coke." *New Statesman*, 29 October 1982.
Dipalma, Joseph R. "Cocaine Abuse and Toxicity." *American Family Practitioner AFP Clinical Pharmacology*, Vol. 24, no. 5. (November 1981).
"Drug Abuse in Sports: Denial Fuels the Problem." *Physician and Sportsmedicine*, April 1982.
"Drug Charge Disputed." *New York Times*, 13 January 1984.
"A Drug Expert Discusses The Hollywood Fad That Makes Some Stars High And Others Dead." *People Weekly*, March 1982.
Durso, Joseph. "Kuhn Bans 4 Players For A Year For Drug Use." *New York Times*, 16 December 1983.
Eller, Carl. "Cocaine Almost Ruined Me." *USA Today*, 11 August 1983.
English, Carey W. "Getting Tough On Worker Abuse Of Drugs, Alcohol." *U.S. News & World Report*, 5 December 1983.
"Ex-Addict Takes It One Day At A Time." *Newsweek*, 23 November 1981.
"Ex-Congressman Was Cocaine User." *New York Post*, 17 January 1984.
Fairbanks, David N.F., and Fairbanks, Grant R. "Cocaine Uses and Abuses." *Annals of Plastic Surgery*, Vol. 10, no. 6 (June 1983).
Falco, Mathea. "The Big Business Of Illicit Drugs." *New York Times Magazine*, 11 December 1983.

"15 Are Charged in Drug Case." *New York Times,* 10 December 1983.

"432 Pounds of Cocaine Is Seized." *New York Times,* 1 December 1983.

"FP Draws Heat For Giving Cocaine To Quell Inflammation." *Medical World News,* 9 July 1979.

Gallo, Bill. "20% Of Active Pros Said To Have Tried It." (N.Y.) *Daily News,* 15 January 1984.

Garber, Phil. "Cocaine Abuse Hotline Brings Stories Of Terror." (N.J.) *Morristown Daily Record,* 10 May 1983.

Gawin, Frank H. "Drugs and Eros: Reflections on Alphrodisiacs." *Journal of Psychedelic Drugs,* Vol. 10, no. 3 (July–September 1978).

Gay, George R. "Cocaine." *Journal of Psychoactive Drugs,* Vol. 13, no. 4 (October–December 1981).

Gay, George R. "You've Come A Long Way, Baby! Coke Time For The New American Lady Of The Eighties." *Journal of Psychoactive Drugs,* Vol. 13, no. 4 (October–December 1981).

Gold, M.S., et al. "Cocaine Withdrawal: Efficacy of Tyrosine." *Society for Neuroscience Abstracts,* 6–11 November 1983.

———Interviews and Direct Communications. Mimeographed. Fall 1983–Winter 1984.

———*Neuropsychopharmacology of Cocaine*. Fair Oaks Hospital, Summit, N.J., 1984.

———*Questions About Cocaine and Its Abuse*. Pamphlet. 800-COCAINE, Fair Oaks Hospital, Summit, N.J., 1983.

Gold, Mark S., and Annitto, William J. *Do You Know The Facts About Drugs?* Hollywood, Florida: Health Communications, Inc., 1983.

Gold, Mark S., and Verebey, K. "Psycholpharmacology of Cocaine." In *Psychiatric Annals on Cocaine,* edited by M.S. Gold. Thorofare, N.J.: Slack Inc., 1984.

Grinspoon, Lester, and Bakalar, James B. *Cocaine: A Drug and Its Social Evolution*. New York: Basic Books, Inc., 1976.

Harmetz, Aljean. "Hollywood Takes Steps To Combat Drug Abuse." *New York Times,* 21 March 1984.

Helfrich, Antionette Ander; Crowley, Thomas J.; Atkinson, Carol A.; and Post, Robin Dee. "A Clinical Profile of 136 Cocaine Abusers." *NIDA Research Monograph Se-*

ries, *Problems of Drug Dependence, 1982*, April 1983.
"How Drugs Sap The Nation's Strength." *U.S. News & World Report*, 16 May 1983.
"Is Show Biz Pushing Drugs? The Big Debate." *U.S. News & World Report*, 16 May 1983.
"Jodie Foster Charged In Cocaine Case." *New York Times*, 29 December 1983.
Johnson, Roy S. "A Compromise on Richardson." *New York Times*, 25 December 1983.
———"Richardson Reinstated By The Nets." *New York Times*, 22 December 1983.
———"Richardson Says Addiction Is Cured." *New York Times*, 14 June 1983.
Junior, E.J. "'I'm kind of glad I was arrested.'" *USA Today*, 11 August 1983.
Kohn, Howard. "Cocaine: You Can Bank On It." *Esquire*, October 1983.
Krupnick, Jerry. "Mackenzie Phillips, 'One Day At A Time' Return Is Giant Step On Road To Recovery." (Newark, N.J.) *The Star Ledger*, 8 November 1981.
"Kuhn Delays Review." *New York Times*, 21 December 1983.
"Lawyer Indicted In $275,000 Theft." *New York Times*, 11 January 1984.
Lee, David. *The Cocaine Handbook: An Essential Reference*. Berkeley, California: And/Or Press, Inc., 1981.
Lombardi, John. "A Lethal Drug Cocktail." (N.Y.) *Daily News*, 29 April 1984.
"Mackenzie Phillips And Her Rock Legend Dad Toil To Escape The Rack Of Drugs." *People Weekly*, 2 March 1981.
Madden, Bill. "Rose's Arm Liability." (N.Y.) *Daily News*, 15 January 1984.
Martin, Everet G. "High Drama: In The Jungles Of Peru, Fight Against Cocaine Is A Tangled-Up Affair. *The Wall Street Journal*, 20 March 1984.
Mehr, Martin. "Companies Coax Drug, Alcohol Problems Out." *The Financial Post*, 10 July 1982.
Menaker, Drusie. "New Drug Aids Addicted Doctors." (Wilmington, Delaware) *Evening Journal*, 17 May 1982.
"Miss Foster May Be Charged With Possession Of Cocaine." *New York Times*, 21 December 1983.
Narvaez, Alfonso A. "Cocaine Hot Line Draws A Thousand Calls A Day." *New York Times*, 1 June 1983.

Ng, David. "20 Seized In Huge B'klyn Cocaine Sweep," *New York Post,* 22 December 1983.
Ondrejas, Carolyn. "Cocaine: A Dangerous Seduction." *Fort Worth Star-Telegram,* 15 November 1981.
"1,600 Pounds Of Cocaine Seized In Van In Queens." *New York Times,* 17 December 1983.
Penn, Stanley. "Columbia's Drug Kings Move Freely." *The Wall Street Journal,* 28 November 1983.
Penn, Stanley, and Pound, Edward T. "Havana Haven: Smugglers Of Drugs From Columbia To U.S. Are Protected By Cuba." *The Wall Street Journal,* 30 April 1984.
Perry, David. "The Pharmacology of Addiction and Drug Dependence." *PharmChem Newsletter,* July 1976.
Petersen, Robert C., et al. *Cocaine: A Second Look.* The American Council on Marijuana and Other Psychoactive Drugs, Inc., 1983.
Pileggi, Nicholas. "There's No Business Like Drug Business." *New York Magazine,* 13 December 1982.
"Pitcher Denied Bail." *New York Times,* 12 January 1984.
Plowman, Timothy. "Botanical Perspectives on Coca." *Journal of Psychedelic Drugs,* Vol. 11, no. 1–2 (January–June 1979).
Pope, Jr., Harrison G.; Ionescue-Pioggia, Martin; and Cole, Jonathan O. "Drug Use and Life-style Among College Undergraduates." *Archives of General Psychiatry,* May 1981.
"Pryor Pleads Not Guilty In Drug Case." *New York Times,* 30 December 1983.
Pursch, Joseph. "The Western World's Most Dangerous Drug." *USA Today,* 11 August 1983.
Rasky, Susan. "U.S. Seizes Eastern Jetliner Carrying Cocaine." *New York Times,* 25 April 1984.
Reel, Bill. "Her—A Junkie?" (N.Y.) *Daily News,* 18 December 1983.
"Richardson Ready." *New York Times,* 27 December 1983.
Riding, Alan. "Colombia Starts Huge Drug Drive." *New York Times,* 12 May 1984.
Rosen, Bruce. "On The American Dream's Dark Side." (Bergen County, N.J.) *Sunday Record,* 14 March 1982.
Sansweet, Stephen J.; Petzenger, Jr., Thomas; and Putka, Gary. "High Fliers: Use Of Cocaine Grows Among Top Traders In Financial Centers." *Wall Street Journal,* 12 September 1983.

Schmeck, Jr., Harold M. "Drug Abuse In America: Widening Array Brings New Perils." *New York Times*, 22 March 1983.

Semon, Nancy. "Horrors Of Drug Abuse Described By John And Mackenzie Phillips," (Westfield, N.J.) *Suburban News*, 8 April 1981.

"Sequel." *People Weekly*, Vol. 16, no. 26 (December 1981–January 1982).

Seymour, Richard. Interviews and Direct Communications. Haight-Ashbury Free Medical Clinic, San Francisco, Winter 1983.

Shriver, Jerry. "Employers Are Helping Addicted Workers: Coke Lures A 'New Class'; The Signs Of Abuse." *USA Today*, 12 January 1984.

Siegel, Ronald. "History of Cocaine Smoking." *Journal of Psychoactive Drugs*, Vol. 14, no. 4 (October–December 1982).

———"Cocaine Substitutes." *PharmChem Newsletter*, July–August 1982.

"Sitzberger Is Linked To Coast Cocaine Case." *New York Times*, 7 January 1984.

Smart, Reginald G., Liban, Carolyn, and Brown, Geoff. "Cocaine Use Among Adults And Students." *Canadian Journal of Public Health*, Vol. 72 (November/December 1981).

Smight, Tim. "Getting Straight: Mackenzie Phillips Talks About The Dangers Of Addiction As She Battles Her Own Drug Habit—One Day At A Time." *Sourcebook, The Magazine For Seniors*, 1982.

Smith, David E. "Cocaine Abuse." Paper presented at the Women and Work Conference, November 1982, New York City.

———Interviews and Direct Communications. Haight-Ashbury Free Medical Clinic, San Francisco, Spring 1981–Winter 1983.

———"Abuse Folio." *High Times*, February 1984.

Smith, David E., and Wesson, Donald R. "Cocaine." *Journal of Psychedelic Drugs*, Vol. 10, no. 4 (October–December 1978).

———"Consideration of Cocaine Dosage." *Journal of Psychedelic Drugs*, Vol. 10, no. 4 (October–December 1978).

Span, Paula. "Treating The Affluent Drug Addict." *USA Today*, 9 January 1984.

"State Lax In Fight On Cocaine Addiction." *New York Times*, 11 December 1983.

Steyer, Robert. "Drug Finds A New Use Easing Withdrawal Symptoms." (Newark, N.J.) *Sunday Star-Ledger*, 16 March 1980.

Stripp, David. "Open Mind: Mysteries Of The Brain Slowly Yield To Science, And Medicine Benefits." *Wall Street Journal*, 19 December 1983.

"Strung Out And Calling It Quits." *Time*, 23 May 1983.

Stuart, Reginald. "Court Bars Data On Kennedy Death." *New York Times*, 4 May 1984.

"Taking Drugs On The Job." *Newsweek*, 22 August 1983.

Talan, Jamie. "New Drug Proposed For Treating Addicts." *New York Times*, 29 November 1983.

"Teacher Arrested As Cocaine Seller." *New York Times*, 7 January 1984.

Tennant, Jr., Forest S,. and Rawson, Richard A. "Cocaine and Amphetamine Dependence Treated With Desipramine." *NIDA Research Monograph Series, Problems of Drug Dependence*, April 1983.

Van Dyke, Craig, and Byck, Robert. "Cocaine." *Scientific American*, Vol. 246, no. 3 (March 1982).

Verebey, K., and Gold, M.S. "Psychopharmacology of Cocaine: Behavior, Neurophysiology, Neurochemistry and Proposed Treatments." In *Psychopharmacology: Impact On Clinical Psychiatry*, edited by B.W. Morgan. St. Louis: Ishiyaku EuroAmerica, Inc.

Weissman, J.C. "Understanding the Drugs and Crime Connection." *Journal of Psychedelic Drugs*, Vol. 10, no. 3 (July–September 1978).

Wetli, Charles V., and Wright, Ronald K. "Death Caused by Recreational Cocaine Use." *Journal of American Medical Association*, Vol. 241, no. 23 (8 June 1979).

Werner, Leslie Maitland. "Drug War Is Mainly A 'Holding Action.'" *New York Times*, 18 December 1983.

Whitlow, Joan. "Cocaine's 'Glamor' Masks Growing Danger." (Newark, N.J.) *Sunday Star-Ledger*, 14 March 1982.

Wilford, B.B. *Drug Abuse: A Guide for the Primary Care Physician*. Chicago: American Medical Association, 1981.

Yang, J.L., et al. Untitled. *Anesthesia and Analgesia*, Vol. 64, no. 4 (April 1982).

DAVID E. SMITH, M.D. is president and medical director of the Haight-Ashbury Free Medical Clinical, which he founded in 1967. He is also associate clinical professor of toxicology, Department of Pharmacology, University of California Medical School at San Francisco. Long regarded as one of the nation's foremost experts on drugs and drug abuse, Dr. Smith has been a consultant to numerous government agencies and medical and health professionals. Recent programs developed by Dr. Smith include treatment and support for addicted physicians and nurses and cocaine support groups for addicted lawyers, stockbrokers, and other professionals. His first priority remains treating destitute drug abusers in the Haight Ashbury.

Dr. Smith and his colleagues have done seminal research on many facets of drug abuse. The treatment protocols he has developed for stimulants, sedative-hypnotics, PCP, and other drugs are now used throughout the world.

His recent areas of research and training include physicians' prescribing practices, lookalike drugs, benzodiazepines, and amphetamines. He is currently involved in developing national drug-prescribing standards.

Founder and editor of the *Journal of Psychoactive Drugs*, Dr. Smith serves on the editorial boards of several professional journals and has written numerous books and articles, including *PCP: Problems and Prevention; Amphetamine Use, Misuse and Abuse; Drugs in the Classroom; Barbiturates: Their Use, Misuse and Abuse;* and *A Multicultural View of Drug Abuse*. With his colleague Richard Seymour, Dr. Smith writes a monthly consumer information column for *High Times*.

RICHARD B. SEYMOUR, M.A., is training director of the Haight-Ashbury Free Medical Clinic and David E. Smith's writing and research associate. As executive administrator, he guided the clinic through the turbulent early 1970s. Mr. Seymour was the first chairman of a statewide California coalition of drug abuse treatment programs and is the current chairperson of the Marin County (California) Drug Abuse Advisory Board. He has been instrumental in the development of physician- and nurse-training courses in drug abuse diagnosis and treatment, prevention, and proper prescribing practices.

A graduate of Sonoma State University, Mr. Seymour has a wide academic background in English and journalism, anthropology and philosophy. Before joining Dr. Smith at the clinic, he worked as a newspaper columnist, cofounded an experimental college, and helped plan the California Open College System. A prolific author, he has written many articles and treatment protocols on drug abuse, in addition to four novels, short stories, and two volumes of poetry. With Dr. Smith, he coauthors a monthly consumer information column on drugs.

Under Mr. Seymour's direction, the Haight-Ashbury Training and Education Project serves health care providers, government agencies, and the general public, as well as a growing number of drug treatment leaders and legislators from abroad. Mr. Seymour is currently preparing a position paper on physicians' prescribing practices and developing physicians' drug-training seminars for use in Europe, South America, and the Far East.

INDEX

—A—

—B—

—D—

—E—

—F—

—G—

—H—

—I—

—J—

—K—

—L—

—M—

—N—

—O—

—P—

—Q—

—R—